Physical Examination Procedures for Advanced Nurses and Independent Prescribers

Evidence and rationale

Physical Examination Procedures for Advanced Nurses and Independent Prescribers

Evidence and rationale

Zoë Rawles BN RGN BSc(Hons), Lecturer/Practitioner, Swansea University; Nurse Practitioner and Independent Prescriber, General Practice; Independent Health Care Trainer, HealthTrain, Wales, UK

Beth Griffiths RGN RM BSc(Hons) MSc, Lecturer/Practitioner, Swansea University; Nurse Practitioner and Independent Prescriber, General Practice, Wales, UK

Trudy Alexander RGN SCM BSc(Hons) Nursing Studies BSc(Hons) Nurse Practitioner PGCE, Lecturer/Practitioner, Swansea University; Nurse Practitioner and Independent Prescriber, General Practice, Wales, UK

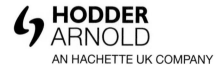

HODDER
ARNOLD
AN HACHETTE UK COMPANY

First published in 2010 by
Hodder Arnold, an imprint of Hodder Education, an Hachette UK Company
338 Euston Road, London NW1 3BH

http://www.hodderarnold.com/

Hachette UK's policy is to use papers that are natural, renewable and recyclable products made from wood grown in sustainable forests. The logging and manufacturing processes are expected to conform to the environmental regulations of the country of origin.

Whilst the advice and information in this book are believed to be true and accurate at the date of going to press, neither the authors nor the publisher can accept any legal responsibility or liability for any errors or omissions that may be made. In particular (but without limiting the generality of the preceding disclaimer) every effort has been made to check drug dosages; however it is still possible that errors have been missed. Furthermore, dosage schedules are constantly being revised and new side-effects recognized. For these reasons the reader is strongly urged to consult the drug companies' printed instructions before administering any of the drugs recommended in this book.

British Library Cataloguing in Publication Data
A catalogue record for this book is available from the British Library

Library of Congress Cataloging-in-Publication Data
A catalog record for this book is available from the Library of Congress

ISBN   978 0 340 967 584

2 3 4 5 6 7 8 9 10

Commissioning Editor:	Naomi Wilkinson
Project Editors:	Joanna Silman and Jane Tod
Production Controller:	Rachel Manguel
Cover Designer:	Laura DeGrasse
Indexer:	Liz Granger

Typeset in 10 on 14pt Minion by Phoenix Photosetting, Chatham, Kent
Printed and bound in Spain

What do you think about this book? Or any other Hodder Arnold title?
Please visit our website: www.hodderarnold.com

CONTENTS

FOREWORD

The acquisition and development of advanced clinical examination skills is a life-long, complex professional activity. To this end, this straightforward clear-cut text takes the developing advanced clinician step by step through the procedures necessary for clinical examination. Written by three experienced Nurse Practitioners who are Lecturer Practitioners at Swansea University, it is grounded in today's most current clinical practice, and founded in a tested programme of education that has for 20 years been in the frontline of developing advanced practitioners.

The book contains a number of chapters based on fundamental principles and systems. Each chapter is carefully structured, introducing principles and practice, providing detailed checklists, detailing the evidence base, and providing working scenarios and case histories based on real life experiences. Readers may use this format by working systematically through the text, or alternatively use the book selectively as they encounter issues in day-to-day practice.

The authors have developed this text in response to their own students' needs, and it may be widely used by nurses, allied health professionals, Independent Prescribers and medical students. It is also a useful resource for those engaged in teaching these skills to prospective advanced practitioners.

The book will help the reader to understand and develop their skills in:

- the rational choice of examination techniques based upon the available evidence
- tailoring the examination to each person's history and characteristics
- interpretation of examination findings
- consideration of examination findings within the context of a complete and holistic history
- reflection upon everyday practice and professional issues.

The authors have all enjoyed putting this text together, and hope that you will enjoy not just reading it, but *using* it! Clinical practice is always challenging, and the practitioner is always learning. This text will be a useful tool for the practitioner in their life-long clinical practice.

Dr David Barton
Academic Lead – Department of Nursing, School of Health Science, Swansea University
Chair of the National Association of Advanced Nursing Practice Educators
2010

PREFACE

In today's health service there is an increasingly diverse range of healthcare professionals. Each one has an important role in improving accessibility and maintaining high standards of healthcare in a service that is so vital to each and every one of us. In seeking to improve healthcare standards, the roles of healthcare professionals are in a constant state of change and expansion. Physical examination skills, diagnosis and prescribing were once the domain of medicine alone, but today many other healthcare professionals can access additional educational courses to enable them to develop these valuable skills and incorporate them into their work with patients. For most of these professionals this expansion in their role is considered to be 'advanced practice'. Currently healthcare professionals who may have undertaken such courses include nurses in advanced practice such as nurse practitioners, midwives, paramedics and pharmacists.

This book is designed primarily as *a supplementary text* and revision aid for students preparing for their final clinical assessment, but it may also be useful for medical students, teachers of physical examination skills and other qualified health professionals. It is assumed that the reader is already fluent in anatomy, physiology, pathology and therapeutics, and has undertaken a recognized course in clinical assessment skills in their area of practice.

Although the consultation process varies depending upon the setting, history taking, physical examination, investigations, differential diagnosis and management are universal. While this book concentrates on the physical examination aspect it is not designed to provide the reader with a description of *how to* perform each examination. It will however help the reader to determine which techniques would be useful depending upon the information that has already been gathered during history taking. As such it should be considered a valuable adjunct to the many other available texts that provide comprehensive descriptions for each technique. The book contains a vast amount of very condensed information and is a solid, general foundation on which healthcare professionals may wish to build and expand, depending on their area of practice.

Although this book concentrates on the rationale for physical examination it must be remembered that competent history taking provides the cornerstone for an accurate differential diagnosis and that clinical decision-making is a skill requiring knowledge and problem-solving skills. Many good texts, such as one by Tierney and Henderson (2005), deal comprehensively with these subjects.

Health professionals working at an advanced level will be aware of the many professional and ethical issues surrounding their practice. Often these issues are not clear cut when applied to the workplace. For this reason they have been presented as reflections on everyday practice. This will remind the reader of their importance and the need for structured reflection as a tool to unravel some of these problems and promote good quality care.

Special features of this book include the following.

- Unique, evidence-based physical examination procedure lists for each anatomical system. Where necessary concise descriptions of techniques are provided as an aide-memoire. The procedures listed are those that are best supported by the available evidence.

- Comprehensive but concise lists of 'rationale and possible pathology' for the examination procedures. These are linked with the procedures by placing them in the adjacent column which enables the reader to associate quickly underpinning theory with practice. It also encourages the reader to use their reasoning skills to differentiate between examination techniques that may or may not be useful to include in the examination, depending upon the history provided by the patient. Common and significant pathologies have been included in the lists.
- A tabular format for the examination procedure lists, making them easy to use in practice.
- Referral to other chapters for further information where necessary. This emphasizes the need to consider integrated examinations as pathological signs may be found in one or more anatomical systems.
- A chapter on mental health. Although this may not be considered as part of the physical examination, it was deemed necessary as it is often closely entwined in the presentation of physical symptoms. The format of this chapter differs from the previous chapters to enable the reader to distinguish serious mental health issues from somatization of symptoms.
- A discussion of the available evidence and its application to practice in each chapter. This can be cross-referenced to some of the procedures found in the tables.

    A thorough search was undertaken for good-quality research in order to rationalize the various procedures and techniques traditionally used in physical examination where methods ad infinitum exist, to the bewilderment of the fledgling practitioner.

    The reference list inevitably contains older, smaller studies when larger, more recent studies have not been carried out. Seminal journal articles and good-quality reviews of evidence are included.
- Reflection on practice presented as stories illustrating a wide range of professional and ethical dilemmas that may be encountered by professionals practicing at an advanced level. These are based upon the authors' personal reflections from many years of clinical practice in primary care. All names and identifying features have been changed to protect anonymity. This again serves to link underlying theoretical principals and everyday practice.
- Case studies relating to the subject matter of the chapter with short test questions that allow the reader to evaluate their diagnostic reasoning and underpinning knowledge. The case studies can be adapted to any setting where the patient presents with an undiagnosed condition.

The combination of these features helps the reader to integrate theory into everyday practice, while providing an aide-memoire for use in practice or revision for exams.

Evidence-based practice has been the byword of every good clinician for a number of years. Good-quality research is considered to be vital in the decision-making process, but it must be tailored to the individual patient and cannot always eclipse the wealth of tacit knowledge that the experienced practitioner possesses. Such tacit knowledge should not be underestimated. It should be cultivated through reflection and used in conjunction with evidence-based practice.

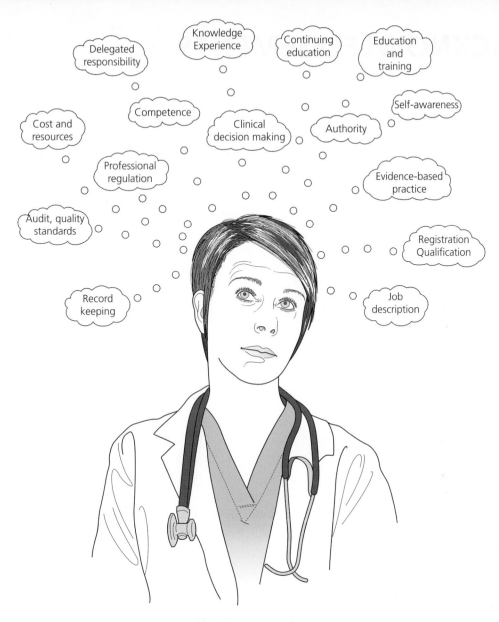

Accountability and clinical practice.

ACKNOWLEDGEMENTS

Thank you to family and friends who supported us in the writing of this book. It has been a long and arduous but ultimately satisfying journey for us all.

Special thanks to Helen Rushford for her help and to Dr David Barton (Swansea University) for words of encouragement!

HOW TO USE THIS BOOK

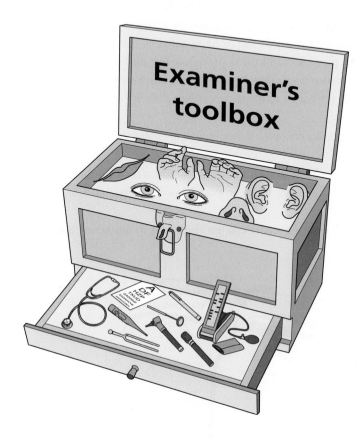

Examiner's toolbox.

This book is designed for use in a generalist setting and is specifically for adults. It should not be applied to children, babies or pregnant females.

Each chapter, apart from the preliminary examination chapter and the mental health chapter, represents an anatomical system. Examination of the anatomical systems should be preceded by the preliminary examination. The preliminary examination chapter illustrates the many signs that may be elicited from this examination alone.

Within each chapter there is a table containing a list of physical examination procedures, each of which is linked to relevant examples of possible pathology or rationale in the adjacent column. After a full history has been taken the health professional will have formulated provisional differential diagnoses. At this stage verification is sought through physical examination for signs of these diagnoses. The tables will help the health professional to determine which examination techniques may be useful in eliciting those signs and to consider other diagnostic possibilities. The reader is therefore encouraged to choose the most relevant procedures from the list. The list of possible pathologies is comprehensive but not exhaustive.

It will often be necessary to integrate the anatomical system examinations, as many symptoms have multiple possible causes which produce signs in one or more systems. The reader is referred to other chapters as appropriate. For example, a problem with the lower limb may require musculoskeletal, neurological and cardiac elements in the examination. Likewise a patient presenting with chest pain may require elements of a cardiac, abdominal and musculoskeletal examination. The reader will need to decide which procedures are necessary and can use the tables to help guide their decision-making.

Where there is evidence key words will be highlighted in green text with a magnifying glass icon in the margin beside the physical examination procedure list; this will give a page number to go to where a discussion of the evidence can be found under the relevant heading in the evidence section of the same chapter. This will help the reader to decide upon the reliability of findings when making a differential diagnosis.

Text that appears in *italics* denotes information supplementary to the core text that the clinician may find useful in practice.

Reflective stories are included in each chapter to demonstrate the difficulties encountered in everyday practice and to remind the reader of the important professional and ethical issues surrounding their work.

At the end of each chapter the reader can test their skills by answering questions pertaining to a case study.

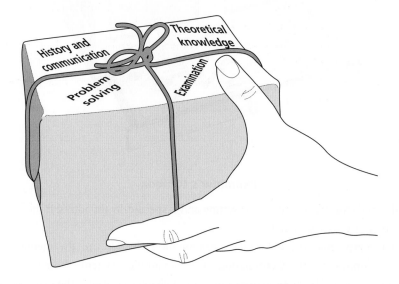

The practitioner skills package.

1 THE PRELIMINARY EXAMINATION

Zoë Rawles

The preliminary examination is the first step in the physical examination and serves to initiate physical contact and reassure the anxious patient. It also begins the process of building up a complete picture of the patient. It should precede all specific examinations and its importance cannot be overestimated as if omitted, then important relevant signs may be missed. For example, there may be a raised blood pressure in an otherwise normal cardiac examination, an enlarged (hyperactive) thyroid gland may provide the clue to an underlying cause for an arrhythmia, or a rash may be an indicator for an autoimmune disease. There may be signs of anaemia that indicate the need for further investigations or there may be oedema signifying cardiac or renal disease. The preliminary examination may also guide the practitioner to a specific examination. An example of this is where the detection of an irregular pulse will dictate the need for a full cardiac examination.

Most of the checks recommended in the procedure list are determined by the need to identify well-recognized pathological findings.

Ensure that the patient is warm and comfortable and that the environment is private as discomfort or anxiety may affect the vital signs.

CHECKLIST

PROCEDURE	RATIONALE/POSSIBLE PATHOLOGY
Assess the general condition of the patient. Assess whether comfortable or distressed, well hydrated, well nourished. Observe physique, gait, mobility, mental capacity, attitude, facial expression and complexion, clothing, level of cleanliness, odour	This builds up a picture of the patient's general health and possible contributory factors to the presenting complaint
Assess whether you can proceed with the examination without causing unnecessary distress or delay	
Look for any obvious sign or recognizable condition or pathology	For example: Cyanosis Jaundice Down's syndrome (*may be associated with various pathologies including congenital heart disease, coeliac disease, Alzheimer's disease*)

Checklist continued

	Cachexia (*signs of obvious weight loss and deteriorating physical condition*)
	Marfan's syndrome (*patients are typically tall with long, thin fingers. It is a genetic disorder of the connective tissue associated with heart valve and aortic defects, lung pathology, problems with eyes and skeleton*)
	Bilateral exophthalmos (*abnormal protrusion of the eyes typically associated with Graves' disease*)
START WITH THE HANDS **Inspect both hands** Fig. 1.1 shows some of the signs outlined below **Assess temperature**	This makes contact with the patient and can be reassuring while obtaining essential clinical information
• Abnormally cold	Hypothermia
• Localized cool areas	Impaired circulation, e.g. peripheral vascular disease or Raynaud's disease (*reduction of blood supply to fingers or toes when exposed to cold or stress. Extremities become pale or white*)
• Abnormally hot, sweaty or moist skin	Anxiety Exertion Pyrexia Liver disease Obesity Hyperthyroidism Hyperhidrosis (*abnormally excessive perspiration*)
• Clamminess	Acute coronary syndrome Myocardial infarction
• Localized hot areas	Inflammation or infection

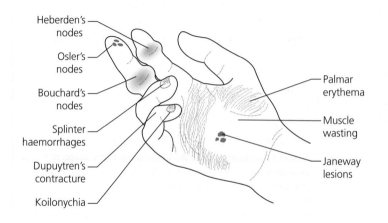

Fig. 1.1. Clinical signs on the hand.

Heberden's nodes
Osler's nodes
Bouchard's nodes
Splinter haemorrhages
Dupuytren's contracture
Koilonychia
Palmar erythema
Muscle wasting
Janeway lesions

Checklist continued

Assess texture and skin turgor	
• Very dry skin	Ageing
	Hypothyroidism
	Dermatitis/eczema
• Poor skin turgor	Dehydration
• Tight shiny skin/oedema	Carpal tunnel syndrome (*compression of the median nerve at the wrist causing paraesthesia and weakness in the affected hand*)
	Lymphoedema secondary to malignancy
	Toxaemia of pregnancy
	Fracture/injury
	Premenstrual
	Obesity
	Renal disease
• Thin skin	Ageing
	Medication, e.g. long-term steroids
• Thickened skin	Hypothyroidism
	Manual work
	Eczema
	Psoriasis
Assess the colour	
• Peripheral cyanosis	Low cardiac output
	Arterial disease
	Obstruction such as in Raynaud's disease
	Hypothermia
	Respiratory disease
• Palmar erythema	Liver disease
	Pregnancy
	Oral contraception
Look for finger clubbing	Hereditary
	Pulmonary disease, e.g. lung cancer
	Cardiac disease, e.g. infective endocarditis, Fallot's tetralogy (*congenital cyanotic heart disease with four anatomical abnormalities*)
	Inflammatory bowel disease
	Idiopathic
Assess the condition of the nails	
Look for	
• Pitting	Psoriasis/psoriatic arthropathy
	Alopecia areata (*hair loss causing bald patches on the scalp*) – the nails are affected in a small number of these patients
	Eczema

9

Checklist continued

• Splinter haemorrhages and/or nailfold infarcts	Trauma
	Bacterial endocarditis
	Vasculitis: commonly associated with connective tissue and rheumatological disease
	Malignant melanoma
• Nicotine staining	Cigarette smoking (may conflict with patient history)
• Koilonychia (*'spooning' of nails*)	Iron deficiency anaemia
• Onycholysis (*separation of nail from nailbed distally and laterally*)	Uncommon but may be due to:
	Thyrotoxicosis
	Psoriasis
	Raynaud's disease
	Trauma
	Fungal infection
Look for deformities: Fig. 1.1	
• Heberden's nodes (*bony nodules at terminal phalanges*)	Osteoarthritis
• Swelling of interphalangeal joints and ulnar deviation of fingers	Rheumatoid arthritis
• Osler's nodes and Janeway lesions (*palpable purpura on the extremities*)	Rare sign in bacterial endocarditis
• Dupuytren's contracture (*shortening and thickening of the fibrous tissue in the palm causing flexion deformity of the fingers*)	Familial
	Cirrhosis and alcoholism
	Medication, e.g. anticonvulsant drugs
	Diabetes
• Wasting	
Unilateral of small muscles	Neurological disease
	Pancoast tumour (*apical lung cancer affecting the brachial plexus*)
Bilateral	Normal ageing
	Rheumatoid arthritis
CHECK FOR ASTERIXIS *Asterixis is sometimes called 'metabolic flap': it describes forward flapping of the hand when the arm is extended and the hand dorsi-flexed for 30 seconds. The patient is unable to maintain a fixed posture because of the sudden disappearance of electrical activity in the muscle, so the hands display a coarse flapping tremor*	Respiratory pathology, e.g. hypercapnoea in chronic obstructive pulmonary disease (COPD) Hepatic failure. Asterixis reflects the neurological effects of hepatic encephalopathy

Checklist continued

PALPATE THE RADIAL PULSE • Unilaterally (or bilaterally) for rate, rhythm and volume If there are concerns regarding the circulatory system generally, bilateral assessment of radial pulses and assessment of other pulses is important (refer to Chapter 2)	This may provide important information about the cardiac function and subsequent quality of peripheral perfusion An abnormal pulse may indicate the need to check other pulses and perform a full cardiac examination
CHECK THE TEMPERATURE **Assess for** • Pyrexia	
	Infection
	Immunological disease, e.g. lupus (*an autoimmune connective tissue disease that can affect many different body systems*), sarcoidosis (*a multisystem disorder with formation of small inflammatory nodules or granulomas, usually in lungs or lymph nodes but can affect any organ*)
	Metabolic disorders, e.g. porphyria (*overproduction of porphyrins in the skin or liver leading to neurological or skin problems*)
	Deep vein thrombosis; pulmonary embolus
	Medication
	Malignancy, e.g. renal cancer and leukaemia
	Unknown origin
• Hypothermia	Primary (due to cold environment)
	Secondary, e.g. due to diabetes, malnutrition, hypothyroidism, stroke
MEASURE THE BLOOD PRESSURE Use an approved technique according to national guidelines Check for: • Raised blood pressure For a definite diagnosis of hypertension, accurate and repeated measurement is imperative *Hypertension is an important risk factor for cardiovascular disease, renal and eye disease*	May be acute, due to stress or illness (further readings may be normal) Essential hypertension: unknown cause Secondary hypertension: due to kidney disease, tumours or endocrine disease May also be caused by medication, e.g. steroids, contraceptive pill, hormone replacement therapy (HRT), some anti-rheumatic drugs, non-steroidal anti-inflammatories

Checklist continued

• Low blood pressure (hypotension)	Septicaemia
	Anaphylaxis
	Hypovolaemia
	Post myocardial infarction
	Neurogenic
	Vasodilation due to heat/medication
	Cardiac dysfunction
	Pulmonary embolus
	Postural
EXAMINE THE EYES **Look for** • Yellowing of the sclera due to jaundice (*if circulating bilirubin >35 µmol/L*)	 Haemolytic anaemia Liver disease, e.g. hepatitis, cirrhosis, malignancy, metastases Obstruction of the bile duct Gilbert's syndrome (*hereditary benign disorder in which increased levels of bilirubin cause jaundice*)
• **Conjunctival rim pallor**	Anaemia
• **Senile arcus** (*peripheral corneal opacity*) and **xanthelasma** (*yellow flat plaques around the eyes that are collections of cholesterol*)	May be associated with increased levels of plasma cholesterol and low-density lipoprotein cholesterol, especially if present in younger males
• Dryness or inflammation	May be associated with autoimmune disorders, e.g. systemic lupus erythematosus, rheumatoid arthritis, ulcerative colitis
• Horner's syndrome *Signs on the affected side of the face include ptosis of the upper eyelid, miosis, dilation lag. There may also be enophthalmos (recession of the eyeball), anhidrosis, loss of ciliospinal reflex (dilation of the pupil in response to pain), bloodshot conjunctiva and flushing of the face* Refer to Chapter 12 for other signs related to specific eye pathology	Most cases are benign but it may be iatrogenic Many possible causes, e.g. Cluster headache (*episodic severe one-sided headaches. Attacks occur in clusters that may last for weeks or months followed by periods of remission*) Middle ear infection Trauma May reflect more serious pathology such as apical lung cancer

Checklist continued

EXAMINE THE MOUTH **Look inside and around the mouth and gums for signs of**	
• Angular stomatitis (*painful cracking, erythema in the angle of the lips*)	Iron deficiency anaemia
• Central cyanosis	Hypoxia with respiratory or cardiac disease
• Dry mucous membranes	Dehydration
• Abnormalities of tongue or gums	Deficiency or disease states
• Dental caries/poor dental hygiene	Increased risk of endocarditis
• Koplik's spots (*white spots inside cheeks*)	Pathognomonic of early measles. Useful where the patient presents with a measles-type rash but the diagnosis is uncertain
Refer to the Chapter 4 for other signs related to specific mouth pathology	
EXAMINE THE LYMPH NODES If a node is enlarged or tender, look for a cause **Palpate the lymph nodes in the head and neck:**	Tender nodes may indicate inflammation or infection. Hard fixed nodes are suggestive of malignancy Fig 1.2 shows the position of the nodes and describes possible areas of pathology
• Pre- and post auricular	
• Occipital	
• Tonsillar	
• Submandibular	
• Submental	
• Anterior and posterior cervical chain	
• Supraclavicular	Virchow's node (*a large hard node in the left supraclavicular fossa*) is a significant finding and may indicate abdominal malignancy
• Infraclavicular	
Palpate axillary nodes and others including femoral and inguinal when there is a suspicion of relevant pathology	

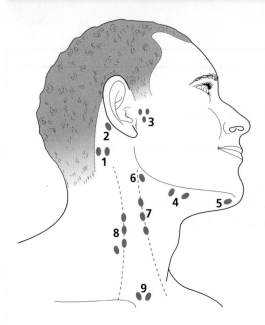

Fig. 1.2. Cervical lymph nodes. Superficial nodes: (1) occipital (draining scalp and skin); (2) post-auricular (scalp and skin); (3) pre-auricular (scalp and skin); (4) submandibular (oral cavity); (5) submental (oral cavity). Deep nodes: (6) tonsillar (tonsillar and posterior pharyngeal regions); (7) anterior – appearing in front of the sternocleidomastoid muscle (larynx, tongue, oropharynx and anterior neck); (8) posterior nodes – appearing behind the muscle (scalp, neck, upper thoracic skin; (9) supraclavicular (gastrointestinal tract, genitourinary tract, pulmonary area).

Checklist continued

EXAMINE THE THYROID GLAND **Observe for visible enlargement** Palpate the thyroid gland from behind the patient with the neck slightly flexed Ask the patient to swallow while your fingers are over the thyroid	The thyroid gland is attached to the trachea and when the patient swallows, both should move upwards. This distinguishes the thyroid gland from other masses which may remain fixed
Note the size, consistency and texture • Enlarged thyroid gland (goitre)	Hashimoto's thyroiditis (*autoimmune disease where the T cells attack the thyroid gland often resulting in hypothyroidism*) De Quervain's thyroiditis (*transient inflammation of the thyroid gland with pain and tenderness. Often characterized by a period of hyperthyroidism followed by transient hypothyroidism*)
• Nodular consistency	Subacute lymphocytic thyroiditis (*'silent throiditis': likely to be autoimmune. Commonly occurs during the post-partum period with symptoms of hyperthyroidism*) Graves' disease (*autoimmune disease causing enlargement of the thyroid gland or goitre and subsequent hyperthyroidism*) Thyroglossal cyst (*usually presents as a fluctuant midline swelling*)

Checklist continued

• Firm/hard texture	Benign tumours, e.g. follicular adenoma, lipoma
	Thyroid carcinoma (papillary and follicular adenocarcinomas)
• Tender with 'woody' texture	Simple goitre
	Hashimoto's thyroiditis
	Malignancy
	Fibrosis
	Cyst
	Calcification
	Acute thyroiditis
AUSCULTATE FOR CAROTID BRUITS (a *turbulent sound*) In patients presenting with syncope, confusion, symptoms of heart disease	May indicate stenosis in the artery
PALPATE FOR PITTING OEDEMA Ankle oedema in the mobile patient or sacral oedema if bed-bound	Occupational /gravitational (prolonged standing)
	Immobility
	Varicose veins
	Heart failure
	Side-effects from some drugs (calcium channel blockers, steroids, non-steroidal anti-inflammatory drugs)
	Decreased oncotic pressure in hepatic, renal and gastrointestinal disease
	Pregnancy
	Post-thrombotic syndrome
	Idiopathic
Now examine a specific system if necessary	

THE EVIDENCE

Radial pulse

There are various techniques for checking the radial pulse. Some practitioners advocate only checking a unilateral radial pulse unless there is known or suspected cardiac or circulatory disease, while others will check bilateral radial pulses simultaneously for every examination. There is no evidence to promote one approach over the other in terms of outcome and so for all examinations other than cardiac, checking a unilateral radial pulse is considered sufficient.

Clubbing

In a review of clinical signs, Karnath (2003) concluded that digital clubbing is a useful clinical sign that may be associated with a number of diseases. While there is little doubt that it is a significant finding, the exact cause for clubbing is still unknown. Various hypotheses have been proposed. Recent research from Leeds University (Uppal *et al.* 2008) suggests a mechanism for clubbing based on high levels of the lipid prostaglandin E2 (PGE2). Patients with a rare form of inherited clubbing were found to have a genetic mutation whereby they fail to produce an enzyme necessary to break down PGE2. Many of the non-inherited disease processes associated with clubbing are also known to result in elevated circulating PGE2 levels.

Osler's nodes and Janeway lesions

Although rare, these are a known pathological phenomenon associated with infective endocarditis (Dalton and Robinson 2001). Osler's nodes are small tender nodules present on the finger or toe pads, and Janeway lesions are small sometimes nodular haemorrhages occurring on the palms or soles. The pathogenesis is as yet unknown and it is difficult to distinguish between the two. Gunson and Oliver (2007) in a dermatopathology presentation of two patients suggest that the clinical appearance may be determined by the anatomical site and recommend further research.

The practitioner should be able to recognize them and their potential significance.

Asterixis

There is little evidence available about the usefulness of asterixis in determining a specific diagnosis as it can be a clue to a number of underlying diseases, but medical opinion indicates that it is useful in determining the severity of disease (Gokula and Khasnis 2003).

Measurement of blood pressure

Current guidelines (developed in accordance with current evidence) for checking blood pressure are available online (NICE 2006b) and include recommendations for best practice. Incorrect technique can have a significant impact on accuracy. An evidence-based review indicates how factors, such as the patient talking or the use of a cuff that is too small, can significantly increase the reading (McAlister and Straus 2001).

The type of device used is also an important factor and the use of portable anaeroid devices as an alternative to those containing mercury is controversial. Tholl *et al.* (2004) in an editorial comment, quote numerous studies and articles suggesting measurement inaccuracy of up to 60 per cent with anaeroid devices with underestimation particularly of the higher readings.

A list of those devices currently considered to be most consistently accurate is available online (British Hypertension Society 2008), but all devices should be regularly calibrated.

Conjunctival rim pallor

This is considered as a compelling indicator of anaemia according to one study where diagnostic accuracy for chronic anaemia as applied to 302 medical and surgical patients was determined (Sheth *et al.* 1997). Patients were prospectively assessed for pallor by at least one of three observers who were not informed of the haemoglobin levels. The presence of conjunctival pallor alone is reason enough to perform a check of haemoglobin. However, the absence of conjunctival rim pallor does not rule out severe anaemia.

Senile arcus and xanthelasma

A systematic review by Fernández *et al.* (2007) concluded that the presence of corneal arcus in a young person indicates the need for further investigation and search for lipid abnormalities

A small-scale study of homozygous familial hypercholesterolaemia patients supports the relationship between the presence of xanthoma or arcus and hypercholesterolaemia with atherosclerosis and recommends further research in this area (Zech and Hoeg 2008).

REFLECTION ON PRACTICE

USING CHECKLISTS THOUGHTFULLY

The student practitioner approached his Objective Structured Clinical Exam (OSCE – final clinical exam) with confidence. He took a history and established that the patient was a heavy smoker who had increasing shortness of breath and fatigue on exertion. For the last 2–3 years, he had a morning cough with grey phlegm. The diagnosis of chronic obstructive pulmonary disease (COPD) seemed obvious. The student performed the examination according to the respiratory checklist, but omitted the preliminary examination and consequently forgot to check the pulse and blood pressure.

During auscultation he put the stethoscope in the correct areas, as he had been taught, but failed to hold it in one position for long enough to assess accurately a full expiration.

To compound these errors further, he was so convinced that this was a straightforward respiratory problem, he failed to appreciate the need for even a cursory examination of the cardiac system.

The patient expressed reservations and asked about possible cardiac pathology. The student however was so intent on remembering his checklist, that the patient's comments were perceived as an unnecessary distraction. He diagnosed likely COPD to be 'confirmed' with spirometry and prescribed inhaled medication.

He also suggested checking a full blood count 'in case of anaemia' and advised his patient on smoking cessation.

Because he was so 'railroaded' and intent on completing his checklist, the student committed many fatal errors and he was failed outright.

- Communication skills suffered and he failed to listen to the patient's concerns.
- He missed a wheeze on expiration because he was 'going through the motions' and not truly listening or connecting his stethoscope with his brain.
- He missed a raised blood pressure of 192/100.
- He missed an irregular heart beat and a tachycardia of 140.

Therefore although the student may have correctly identified one particular problem, he failed to see the complete picture and missed the diagnosis of atrial fibrillation and the raised blood pressure. The subsequent delay in appropriate treatment for this patient may have been very significant.

This type of 'railroading' is a common error, particularly early on in practice. Checklists should be used as an aide-memoire only and should be evidence based where possible. Beware of using checklists as an alternative to thinking.

CASE STUDY

62-year-old male

Presenting complaint: Increasing fatigue and shortness of breath, worse on exertion. He looks pale and unwell.

History of presenting complaint: Symptoms have been coming on over the past few months but recently have become much worse.

Has also had a cough for some years with some grey sputum that is worse in the morning and he attributes this to his smoking history.

Sleeps well on two pillows and does not complain of any pain.

Medical history: Hypertension but no recent checkups.

Drug history: Atenolol 50 mg once daily as prescribed some years ago for hypertension.

Family history: Father died from a myocardial infarction at 59 years. Mother is still alive and well. No siblings and no children.

Social history: Retired salesman. Wife died 2 years ago from a heart attack. Had been married for 35 years. Ex-heavy smoker of 30–40 a day for 40 years (stopped 4 years ago).

continued ➤

CASE STUDY *continued*

Never takes any strenuous exercise.
Plays bowls regularly and drinks about
12 units a week.

Enjoys cooking and his diet is varied with
moderate amounts of fat and plenty of fruit
and vegetables.

Systems review: Usually cheerful but feeling a
little down recently as he cannot do as much as
he used to. Appetite is not so good at the
moment although his weight has been fairly
steady. Nil else of note.

Your preliminary examination reveals a blood
pressure of 172/104 and regular pulse of 52
beats per minute. His body mass index is 28.

Test yourself

1 List the other clinical signs that may be picked
up during the preliminary examination that
indicate the need for a more thorough
examination of the respiratory system.
2 Why would it also be important to examine
the cardiovascular system?
3 Why is the slow pulse rate of significance
here?
4 Assuming the examination of specific systems
is unremarkable, what are your differential
diagnoses at this stage?

Answers to be found at the back of the book
(p. 121).

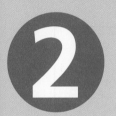

2 THE CARDIOVASCULAR SYSTEM

Beth Griffiths

Examination of the cardiovascular system should include the whole of the circulatory system not just the heart. This chapter starts with particular indicators for cardiac disease then addresses the pulses, the jugular venous pressure (JVP) and proceeds to examination of the chest and heart.

Cardiac risk assessment must be considered as it is useful as a screening tool for treatment purposes. For further reading please go to www.cks.library.nhs.uk/cvd_risk_assessment_and_management.
Perform a preliminary examination first. Pay particular attention to appearance, vital signs, cyanosis, hands, eyes and oedema.

CHECKLIST

PROCEDURE	RATIONALE/POSSIBLE PATHOLOGY
LOOK FOR CLUES OF PRE-EXISTING HEART DISEASE	
• Obesity	Increased cardiac risk
• Cachexia (*weight loss and deterioration in physical condition*)	Common in chronic cardiac failure
• Marfanoid	Risk of aortic valve disease or aortic dissection
• Malar flush	Mitral stenosis or chronic low-output state
• Dysmorphic	
Hypertelorism (*wide-set eyes*)	Could indicate pulmonary stenosis
Elfin facies (*receding jaw, flared nostrils, pointed ears*)	Could indicate supravalvar aortic stenosis
• Down's syndrome (*flat profile, small nose, low-set ears and simian crease*)	Congenital heart defects
PULSE	
Palpate pulses to check for	
• Rate (radial)	
Rate <60 bpm (beats per minute)	Normal for athletes and when sleeping but otherwise could indicate:
	Hypothyroidism
	Heart block
	Hypothermia
	Raised intracranial pressure
	Drug induced

Checklist continued

Rate >120 bpm	Normal during exercise or in anxiety
	Could indicate:
	   Fever
	   Hyperthyroidism
	   Shock due to blood loss or heart failure
	   Drug induced

• Rhythm (radial) Regularly irregular	Missing every few beats, or irregular as in atrial fibrillation or multiple ectopic beats
Irregularly irregular	Atrial fibrillation
Regular with occasional 'dropped beats' (*felt as missed beat followed by exaggerated beat*)	Ectopic beats (*common and usually harmless*)
• Character/volume (carotid) Common abnormalities of **pulse volume and character**:	
• Pulsus alternans: *alternating strong and weak beats*	Severe left ventricular dysfunction (*has less significance if heart rate is rapid*)
• Pulsus biseferiens: *difficult to palpate, 2 beats per cardiac cycle both in systole, sometimes described as slow rising and collapsing pulse*	Aortic regurgitation or a combination of aortic regurgitation and stenosis
• Corrigan pulse, water-hammer: *an abrupt, very rapid upstroke of the peripheral pulse, followed by rapid collapse*	Aortic regurgitation Patent ductus arteriosus Large arteriovenous fistulas Hyperkinetic states Thyrotoxicosis Anaemia Extreme bradycardia
• Pulsus parvus et tardus: *small volume and sharp upstroke pulse*	Aortic stenosis
Familiarity of the carotid pulse is very important for timing of murmurs	These pulse abnormalities are found only when the valve lesion is at least moderately severe
• **Pulsus paradoxus**: *there is a decrease in pulse volume during inspiration in the presence of cardiac tamponade*	Cardiac tamponade
Peripheral pulses Major arteries should be examined to determine the patency of arterial system or if there is evidence of ischaemia in the history	

Checklist continued

Palpate	
• For absence or abnormality	Absence of a limb pulse is often indicative of ischaemia; *the cause is mainly due to atherosclerosis or embolism and it is almost always of significance*
Radial	Aortic aneurysm (refer to Chapter 5)
Brachial	
Abdominal	May be occluded by abdominal tumour
Femoral	
Popliteal	
Dorsalis pedis	Congenitally absent in 2 per cent of patients
Posterior tibial	Congenitally absent in 0.1 per cent of patients
When a pulse is not palpable on a healthy individual, it is usually audible by a **Doppler** flow meter	The **peripheral pulses** may be absent in presence of ischaemia but this alone should not constitute a diagnosis of peripheral vascular disease (PVD)
• For equality	Inequality of the pulses can determine further disease and if ischaemia or limb problems are suspected detailed examination of the peripheral pulses is necessary
Radial: left and right	Aortic dissection proximal to the left subclavian artery or large vessel vasculitis
Femoral: left and right	Occlusion due to an aortic aneurysm may also delay the pulse
	Coarctation of the aorta
• For delay	
Radio-femoral delay	Coarctation of the aorta
	Atheroma
	Inflammatory arteritis in the bilateral iliac arteries or the aorta
Radial-apical deficit	Atrial fibrillation
Auscultate for bruits in major arteries	May be an indication of stenosis in an artery or occur due to turbulence in the flow of blood through the artery
• Carotid bruits	Stenosis, atherosclerosis
• Aortic bruits	Aortic aneurysm
• Renal bruits	Renal artery stenosis
• Popliteal bruits	Aneurysm
*The diagnostic value of **bruits** is now superseded by Doppler examination, but their presence associated with other abnormal findings is very important when diagnosing PVD*	
Buerger's test	
Observation of the colour of the patient's leg when it is elevated and then when it is lowered	Abnormal pallor with elevation and a deep rubor in the lowered position are features of vascular disease

Checklist continued

Venous filling time	
Following elevation of the limb for 1 minute at 45° above supine, it should not take more than 15 seconds for prominent dorsal veins in the foot to refill to above skin level	For use in combination with other markers, in the diagnosis of PVD
JUGULAR VENOUS PRESSURE (JVP) **Check for** • *Height (should be <3 cm above sternal angle)*	
Raised venous pressure if above 3 cm	Heart failure Pulmonary embolus Pericardial effusion Pregnancy Excess intravenous (IV) fluids Liver failure with portal hypertension or pressure from a tumour
• Character and waveforms	Useful for more detailed diagnosis of cardiac abnormalities but no evidence found on reliability only consensus of opinion
• **Hepatojugular reflux:** (**abdominojugular test**) *application of sustained firm pressure over the liver produces a rise in JVP. If the rise in JVP is sustained for longer than 15 seconds it suggests pathology*	All of the above for raised JVP and: Tricuspid regurgitation Heart failure due to other non-valvular causes
• Kussmaul's sign: *(JVP becomes more distended during inspiration, normally decreases on inspiration)*	Constrictive pericarditis Cardiac tamponade Inferior vena cava obstruction Constrictive pericarditis Severe right-sided heart failure Cardiac tamponade Tension pneumothorax
EXAMINATION OF THE PRECORDIUM **Inspect for** • Scars • Deformity • Pulsations • Gynaecomastia **Palpate for** • Heaves: *the apex pushes against the inner rib cage*	Previous surgery Congenital abnormality Chronic respiratory disease Increased heart size May be a side-effect of digoxin or spironolactone Liver disease Ventricular hypertrophy

Checklist continued

• Thrills: *there is a tapping against the inner ribcage; this is always of pathological significance*	Abnormality of the heart valves
• **Apical pulse:** *apex beat should be in fifth intercostal space, midclavicular line, deviation suggests pathology*	Left ventricular dilatation and/or dysfunction. May also be displaced by deformity of chest wall or spine and in chronic lung disease
Auscultate:	
Use bell and diaphragm as diaphragm transmits higher pitched sounds and bell lower pitched sounds	
Apply to the four areas as in Fig. 2.1	
• Listen to heart sounds S1 and S2 for:	
Murmurs noting: location, radiation, timing, pitch, character and intensity	Valvular pathology
Rhythm and rate	Arrhythmias, e.g. atrial fibrillation
Added sounds	Heart failure
S3	S3 can be normal in healthy children or young adults <35 years and pregnant women. It is otherwise pathological and can be due to heart failure, mitral regurgitation or constrictive pericarditis
S4	Indicates a ventricle with decreased compliance so can be normal in older people because of the effects of ageing, but usually pathological
	Ventricular hypertrophy
	Hypertension
Snaps or clicks	Valvular pathology
	Prosthetic heart valves
Pericardial rub	Pericarditis
	Acute myocardial infarction
• Listen to breath sounds	Respiratory pathology (refer to Chapter 3)
	Pulmonary oedema: heart failure

Fig. 2.1. Cardiac heart sounds.

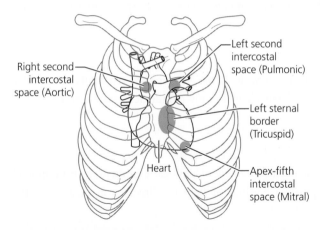

Right second intercostal space (Aortic)

Left second intercostal space (Pulmonic)

Left sternal border (Tricuspid)

Heart

Apex-fifth intercostal space (Mitral)

Checklist continued

Additional check of mitral valve	
Tapping or diastolic rumble may be heard well with bell of the stethoscope in left lateral position	If murmur heard or other clinical findings suggest mitral disease
Additional check of aortic valve	
Sitting forward, a diastolic blowing sound may be accentuated at the end of expiration	If murmur heard or other clinical findings suggest aortic disease
Percussion	
Posterior chest wall for dullness	Respiratory pathology (refer to Chapter 3)
	Pulmonary oedema: heart failure

THE EVIDENCE

The research in this field is mainly limited to cardiac examination performed by cardiologists or specialists in emergency care.

There is wide acknowledgement within the literature of the erosion of clinical skills in cardiovascular examination (Kirby and MacLeod 2006; Shub 2003; Mangione 2001).

Cardiac risk assessment

This is very useful for screening and helps to rationalize the selection of patients for primary prevention strategies. However, in a review of the literature, O'Donnell and Elosua (2008) do not recommend its use for diagnosis as specificity and sensitivity are low.

Volume and character of pulse

Many textbooks describe the assessment of volume and character of the pulse, but there is a lack of evidence to support these as useful signs. Josuha *et al.* (2005) reviewed the evidence and actually advise against relying on the assessment of carotid pulse character. Finlayson *et al.* (1978) describe the various pulse abnormalities as being difficult to recognize, unreliable and contributing nothing to diagnosis, but Babu *et al.* (2003), in a review of evidence, suggest that such signs are not without merit and they recommend an improvement in clinical skills to prevent patients having to be exposed to expensive and time-consuming tests.

Pulsus paradoxus

This has been shown to be the most helpful in diagnosis. It has 98 per cent sensitivity for cardiac tamponade, but is best detected using a blood pressure cuff as only paradoxical pulses exceeding 15–20 mmHg are palpable (McGee 2001).

Peripheral pulses

McGee and Boyko (1998) conducted a detailed critical review of physical examination in peripheral vascular disease and found the following positive findings of help to clinicians in diagnosing the presence of peripheral arterial disease: abnormal pedal pulses, a unilaterally cool extremity, a prolonged **venous filling** time and a femoral **bruit**. Other physical signs help determine the extent and distribution of vascular disease, including an abnormal femoral pulse, lower-extremity **bruits**, warm knees and the Buerger's test. The capillary refill test and the findings of foot discoloration, atrophic skin and hairless extremities are unhelpful in diagnostic decisions (McGee and Boyko 1998).

A systematic review carried out between 1996 and 2005 (United States Preventive Services Task Force 2005) found that in symptomatic patients the most useful findings are the presence of cool skin, the presence of at least one bruit or any palpable pulse abnormality, but clinical findings alone are not independently sufficient to include or exclude a diagnosis of peripheral arterial disease (PAD) with certainty. Khan *et al.* (2006) conducted a systematic review of the evidence and state clearly that the absence of a peripheral pulse is not sufficient for a diagnosis of PAD. The PAD screening score using a hand-held **Doppler** to assess the ankle brachial index (ABI) has much greater diagnostic accuracy (Khan *et al.* 2006) and is now widely recommended.

Buerger's test

In a small but significant study, Buerger's test was found to be a useful adjunct to routine peripheral vascular assessment and a positive finding suggests ischaemia with distal artery involvement (Insall *et al.* 1989). Although the study is old, no further studies have been found and the test is widely recommended for use in practice along with other PAD markers.

The Edinburgh Claudication Score is cited by all of the above and in other papers (original reference: Leng and Fowkes 1992). It has a sensitivity of 91 per cent and a specificity of 99 per cent for the detection of intermittent claudication compared with the physical examination. This reference is also dated but has not been superseded by any others and use of the scoring system in practice is highly recommended, although to date it does not appear to be commonly used.

A meta-analysis conducted by Goodacre *et al.* (2005) states that assessment for **deep vein thrombosis** (DVT) should not be based on individual clinical features. They recommend the use of multiple signs. The use of scores such as Wells' score is highly recommended (Riddle and Wells 2004).

A review of the evidence surrounding Homan's sign conducted by Urbano (2001) states that it is unreliable, insensitive and non-specific in the diagnosis of DVT and it is therefore not recommended for use.

Examination of the peripheral vascular system is useful to assess the patency of the cardiovascular system in total as well as for the diagnosis of peripheral problems. The finding of one abnormality alone is not sufficient for diagnosis but must be used in combination with other findings before a final judgement is made.

Jugular venous pressure

McGee's review in 2001 found good evidence for the clinical value of estimating the jugular venous pressure (JVP). Drazner *et al.* (2001) conducted a large study of 2569 patients that also supports the use of JVP estimation for diagnosis of heart failure. However, no research has been found regarding the assessment of the waveforms although they are commonly quoted in textbooks.

Abdominojugular reflux test (hepatojugular reflux)

This test can be used to detect elevated left and right heart diastolic pressures and it has been found to have a sensitivity of between 55 per cent and 87 per cent and specificity of between 83 per cent and 98 per cent in a review carried out by McGee (2001)

Apical pulse measurement

Deviation of the apical pulse in combination with other signs such as mitral systolic murmur, orthopnoea and hepatomegaly are reliable signs to predict left ventricular dilatation and/or dysfunction with fair sensitivity and excellent specificity (Rovai *et al.* 2007). Although this study was small, two cardiologists correctly diagnosed left ventricular dilatation/dysfunction in 77 per cent of patients after taking a history alone and in 84 per cent of patients after combining history with clinical examination of apical pulse. However, as sensitivity of the test is fair only, the examiner must remember that if the pulse is not deviated this does not rule out a problem.

Auscultation of the heart

This is a complex and difficult skill to acquire and although it is of great value it cannot be taught solely in an academic setting (Kirby and MacLeod 2006). This is an acquired skill that needs to be practised on a regular basis (Joshua *et al.* 2005). There is a lack of robust evidence in the field of heart auscultation particularly concerning the actual placing of the stethoscope with little or no consensus in this area. The placing of the stethoscope varies from a minimum of four positions to a sequence of working inch by inch starting from the apex out into the axilla, back up on the left side of the sternum to the neck and then back down on the right sternal edge to the xiphisternum (Kirby and MacLeod 2006). Positioning of the stethoscope for auscultation in the four areas should not necessarily be directly over the anatomical site. Draper (2008) describes the sites at which the valve sounds may be heard best as follows:

- The mitral valve is best heard at the apex, as this is where the left ventricle is closest to the thoracic cage.
- The tricuspid valve is best heard at the left sternal margin as this is the point closest to the valve where auscultation is possible.
- The pulmonary valve is best heard at the left second intercostal space close to the sternum, where the infundibulum is closest to the thoracic cage.
- The aortic valve is best heard at the right second intercostal space close to the sternum, where the ascending aorta is nearest to the thoracic cage.

These areas will be crucial for detecting abnormalities. Rationale for listening in other areas is lacking in the textbooks and as there is no research evidence to the contrary, the basic four areas of auscultation outlined above are recommended. Most of the more recent studies are focused on new technology and it is anticipated that use of more technologically advanced stethoscopes will allow information to be downloaded to a computer for analysis of the sounds and waveforms. Shub (2003) carried out an extensive review of clinical auscultation versus echocardiography. He concludes that information obtained from auscultation is subjective depending on the examiner's expertise and does not result in a permanent objective recording. It is not readily duplicated by other examiners and its precision for examining systolic murmurs is only fair. Even experienced clinicians disagree about heart sounds and murmurs, but where the clinician is a specialist, the value of auscultation is without doubt. The available research suggests that functional murmurs can be differentiated by clinical examination but accompanying clinical risk assessment and the identification of other signs and symptoms are crucial to achieve a more accurate diagnosis (Shub 2003).

There is not enough evidence assessing the reliability of clinical examinations in primary care. It is therefore recommended that for general clinicians without specialist knowledge or skills, auscultation should not be used without further clinical evaluation if necessary and any diagnosis should be confirmed by an echocardiograph or the patient should be referred to a specialist (Reichlin *et al.* 2004; Shub 2003; Choudhry and Etchells 1999).

 REFLECTION ON PRACTICE

REVIEWING THE DIAGNOSIS
A 75-year-old woman presented in an acute appointment with a history of persistent cough. She had been treated for a respiratory infection initially, then with steroids and a salbutamol inhaler to relieve her symptoms of wheeze and persistent cough. A chest X-ray had been done but the result was not yet available; echocardiograph was ordered but no appointment yet.

Mrs T was very anxious regarding her symptoms and she had a history of anxiety. After taking the history of the 6-week cough, it was obvious that previous attempts at diagnosis and treatment were not fruitful so a full integrated examination was carried out.

Preliminary examination was unremarkable, vital signs and oxygen saturation were within normal limits. Carotid pulse revealed small volume with a blunt upstroke, no bruits. JVP was raised two finger breadths above the manubriosternal angle at 45° supine. There was an ejection (mid) systolic murmur grade III, heard loudest over the aortic area. There were persistent fine crepitations in both lung bases, otherwise respiratory examination was normal.

There was no history of cardiac or respiratory diseases and risk factors for cardiac disease were low; non-smoker, minimal alcohol, body mass index was 26, no record of cholesterol and normal blood pressure.

The significance of this story is to highlight the following points:

- if an integrated examination had been carried out initially she may have been spared taking the antibiotics, steroids and the salbutamol
- being alert to therapy failure is an important point – first one should check compliance, and second one should check the diagnosis
- although the outcome for this lady's case will ultimately be the same, referral may have been made sooner to the cardiologist for further treatment
- although risk factors for cardiac disease are low, the presenting complaint can take many forms.

 CASE STUDY

78-year-old female

Presenting complaint: Loss of power in her left hand for less than 1 hour on 2 occasions.

History of presenting complaint: Came back from weekend in Brighton last night. Three days ago lost the use of her left hand for around 20 minutes; thought it was due to carrying a heavy bag during the morning. It happened again yesterday and she could not identify any cause. Her arm and hand felt cold and weak, nearly dropped the tea cup and was unable to finish her drink. It took about an hour to come back to normal.

No headache, dizziness or facial weakness.
No confusion, dysarthria, loss of memory or abnormal behaviour.
No loss of power in legs. Gait was normal.
No other neurological symptoms.

Past medical history: Nil of note.

Family history: Father died aged 84 years from cerebrovascular accident (CVA), mother died from heart attack aged 83 years. Younger sister and brother, both in good health.

continued ➢

CASE STUDY *continued*

Social history: Widowed 1 year ago now living alone.
  Never smoked but husband did all his life.
  Alcohol – rarely.
  Until now fit and well and living independently, good social network of friends.

Medication: Nil, no recreational or over-the-counter medicines.

Allergies: None known.

Systems review: Recently experiencing palpitations and some shortness of breath.
  No chest pain.
  Sleeps on two pillows.
  No other chest symptoms.
  Sleeps well, appetite good, nil else of note.

Preliminary examination

Pulse is irregular and 105 bpm.
Respirations: 22 per minute.
Temperature: normal.
Blood pressure: 180/100.
No ankle oedema.
Body mass index: 26.

Test yourself

1 What are your differential diagnoses at this stage and which aspects of the history relate to each of these differential diagnoses?
2 What is the significance of the signs found on preliminary examination in this case and how do they help to determine the most likely diagnosis?
3 What specific examinations should be carried out for this lady?
4 What are the main components of this lady's management plan?

Answers can be found at the back of the book (p. 121).

3 THE RESPIRATORY SYSTEM

Zoë Rawles

This checklist identifies the essential components of the respiratory examination.

The patient should be lying at 45° with the chest and back fully exposed. Examine the anterior chest first and then the posterior chest, as this involves less movement for the patient in a potentially tiring examination.

Perform a thorough preliminary examination first (Chapter 1). Pay particular attention to the respiratory rate and the patient's ability to talk in complete sentences. If either of these is abnormal they may be important indicators of respiratory distress.

CHECKLIST

PROCEDURE	RATIONALE/POSSIBLE PATHOLOGY
ANTERIOR CHEST	
OBSERVE **Assess for**	
• Pectus excavatum (*a congenital abnormality where some ribs and the sternum grow abnormally, resulting in a sunken appearance*)	May impair respiratory function
• Abnormal movement or use of accessory muscles	Chronic obstructive pulmonary disease (COPD) Acute or poorly controlled asthma
• Intercostal recession (*drawing in of intercostal spaces during inspiration*)	Indicates severe obstruction of the airways with negative intrathoracic pressure and a non-compliant lung
• Scars	Trauma or surgery
• Parasternal heave	Right-sided ventricular hypertrophy/pulmonary hypertension
• Hyperinflation	COPD with premature airway closure
• Prominent, dilated veins	Commonest cause is mediastinal pressure causing obstruction of the superior vena cava Many possible causes, including bronchial carcinoma, aortic aneurysm, goitre

Checklist continued

Look at how the patient is breathing, the rate depth, pattern	
• Tachypnoea (*more than 25 breaths per minute*)	Hyperventilation, e.g. with anxiety or in response to metabolic acidosis
	Respiratory distress, e.g. in
	Acute asthma attack
	Pulmonary embolism
	Pneumothorax
	Pneumonia (**Can pneumonia be diagnosed from clinical signs alone?**)
• Bradypnoea (<12 breaths per minute)	Neurological disorders
	Medication, e.g. opiates
• Altered pattern of breathing, e.g. Cheyne–Stokes (*periodic breathing in the form of cycles of respiration where breathing is increasingly deeper and then shallower. There may be periods of apnoea*)	Heart failure
	Post-cerebrovascular accident
	Brain tumour
	After the administration of morphine
	Can be normal in sleep
Kussmaul (*deep sighing breathing*)	Associated with metabolic acidosis e.g. in diabetic ketoacidosis or renal failure
Look at the right side of the neck for signs of	
Raised jugular venous pressure (JVP). *The height is usually less than 3 cm*	Superior vena cava obstruction
Refer to Chapter 2 for more information	Cor pulmonale (*right ventricular hypertrophy that occurs in response to increased pressure caused by respiratory disease*)
PALPATE	
• For any **tenderness over chest wall**	Musculoskeletal problem, e.g. fractured rib, costochondritis (*inflammation of the cartilages in the ribcage*)
	Note that the presence of tenderness does not exclude the possibility of other pathology, e.g. pulmonary embolus or co-existent ischaemic heart disease
• Position of trachea (*should be midline*)	In combination with palpation, percussion and auscultation, this is useful to interpret ipsilateral (*same side*) and contralateral (*other side*) mediastinal shifts. Deviation of the trachea may occur: towards an area of collapse or fibrosis or away from a large pneumothorax or pleural effusion
• Apex beat of heart. If palpable, check for displacement	Indicates displacement or distortion of the mediastinum, e.g. in
	Ventricular hypertrophy
	Pneumothorax

Checklist continued

• For symmetrical expansion on the lower chest wall, i.e. the **xiphoid site**	Reduced expansion on one side may indicate: Pneumothorax Collapse Consolidation Effusion
Palpation for **tactile fremitus** (*palpable vibration felt on the chest wall during low frequency vocalization, when the patient is asked to repeat a phrase such as '99'*). May be done at the practitioner's discretion although evidence for its inclusion in routine examination is controversial	May be increased over areas of consolidation and decreased or absent over a pneumothorax or pleural effusion
PERCUSS **Over all areas of lung (Fig 3.1). Note any** • Hyper-resonance • Dullness • Stony dullness	Note that normal percussion does not confirm the absence of significant pathology Hyperinflation Pneumothorax Collapse of airways Localized fibrosis Consolidation such as in pneumonia Effusion
AUSCULTATE Use the **diaphragm of the stethoscope** **Lungs: (Fig. 3.1) Auscultate the same areas as for percussion listening for** • Quality of breath sounds, e.g. bronchial or vesicular	Bronchial sounds anywhere other than over the manubrium may indicate: Consolidation Collapse Fibrosis

The magnifying glass icons in the left margin are labelled (top to bottom): 29, 28, 29, 29.

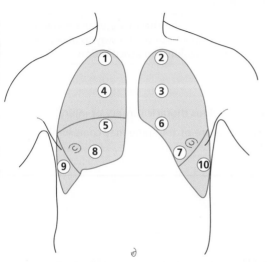

Fig. 3.1. Percussion and auscultation areas on the anterior chest.

Checklist continued

• Adventitious sounds (*added sounds*)	
Crackles	Infection
	Pulmonary congestion
Wheeze	Asthma
	COPD
	Infection
	The duration of wheeze through the respiratory cycle may correspond to the degree of airflow limitation
Rub	Pleurisy
• Diminished/reduced intensity breath sounds	Severe asthma
	Pneumothorax
	Pleural effusion
	Collapse of a major bronchus
Auscultation for vocal fremitus (see tactile fremitus) or whispered pectoriloquy (*perception of the whispered voice during auscultation*) may be done at the practitioner's discretion although as with tactile fremitus, evidence for its inclusion in routine examination is controversial	May be increased over areas of consolidation and decreased or absent over a pneumothorax or pleural effusion
Heart	
Auscultate over atrial, pulmonary, tricuspid and mitral valve areas, to detect abnormal rhythms or murmurs	To detect a cardiac cause for respiratory symptoms:
	Murmurs (may indicate valve stenosis)
Use the bell of the stethoscope over the mitral valve	Arrhythmias, e.g.
	Gallop rhythm (suggestive of heart failure)
	Atrial fibrillation
Abnormal heart sounds or arrhythmias indicate the need for a full cardiac examination (refer to Chapter 2)	
POSTERIOR CHEST	
Ask patient to fold arms across chest	Folding the arms over the chest rotates the scapulae anteriorly moving them out of the way to allow for more sensitive percussion and auscultation
OBSERVE **Look for**	
• Scars	Evidence of previous thoracic surgery or injury
• Deformities, e.g. scoliosis	Abnormal curvature of the spine may compromise respiration

Checklist continued

PALPATE	
• For any **chest wall tenderness**	
• For symmetrical expansion	As for anterior chest

PERCUSS	
• Over all areas of lung (Fig. 3.2)	As for anterior chest
• Over lower chest wall to detect diaphragmatic paralysis or weakness *if indicated, e.g. if patient demonstrates paradoxical inward movement of abdomen during breathing or is dyspnoeic on exertion or has orthopnoea that cannot be explained by other pathology* (*Normal range of movement of diaphragm 5–6 cm*)	Lesions adjacent to phrenic nerve Surgical or other trauma Herpes zoster Cervical spondylosis (*degeneration of the discs and vertebrae in the cervical spine – usually age related*) Idiopathic Recent open heart surgery
AUSCULTATE Lungs: same areas as for **percussion** (Fig. 3.2) **Listen for** • Quality of breath sounds • Adventitious sounds • Diminished/reduced intensity breath sounds	Bronchial breathing is abnormal in posterior or lateral chest and may indicate consolidation or effusion Others as for anterior chest

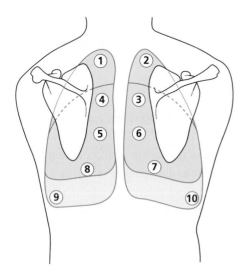

Fig. 3.2. Percussion and auscultation areas on the posterior chest (arms are folded to rotate scapulae anteriorly). Positions 9 and 10 are indicated where the lungs are inflated.

THE EVIDENCE

Several of the references in this section are more than 10 years old. This is regrettable but unavoidable as up-to-date evidence for the usefulness of the various techniques and components of the respiratory examination in predicting pulmonary disease or in distinguishing between the different pathologies is still relatively scarce.

Obstruction of the superior vena cava

Rice *et al.* (2006) reviewed the aetiology and outcome of 78 patients with superior vena cava (SVC) syndrome and identified malignancy in 60 per cent of cases, with bronchogenic carcinoma as the most common form. Twenty-two per cent of the malignancies were due to small cell lung cancer and 24 per cent due to non-small cell lung cancer. The presence of dilated veins on the chest wall, as a possible indicator of SVC obstruction, is therefore significant.

Tactile and vocal fremitus

A review of some studies on procedures traditionally taught in respiratory examination concludes that while auscultation, percussion and vital signs are important, the relevance of techniques such as fremitus and whispered pectoriloquy is less clear (Frank 2006).

Discussion between medical colleagues often reveals incredulity regarding the inclusion of such procedures in the examination, and anecdotally it would seem that these procedures are rarely, if ever, performed other than in objective structured clinical examinations (commonly called OSCEs and referring to the final exams in Nurse Practitioner or independent prescribing courses or in medical training). Therefore, in accordance with the available literature and evidence that questions the usefulness of procedures such as those mentioned, it is suggested that they should only be done at the practitioner's discretion.

Perhaps such procedures should be included in teaching the history of medicine as they have undoubtedly been useful in the past and may continue to be so for those practitioners who wish to specialize in respiratory medicine or for those who intend to practise in areas where modern technology is less readily available.

Respiratory rate

Cretikos *et al.* (2008) report substantial evidence that an abnormal respiratory rate is a predictor of potentially serious clinical events.

The British Thoracic Society (BTS) guidelines for evaluation of the patient with community-acquired pneumonia (2001) support the measurement of respiratory rate as a diagnostic as well as a prognostic tool. They describe a respiratory rate of more than 30 breaths per minute as one of several factors associated with increased mortality, and as such consider it valuable for patient assessment.

A respiratory rate of greater than or equal to 25 breaths per minute in an adult is used as one component of diagnosis in acute severe asthma (Scottish Intercollegiate Guidelines Network [SIGN] and BTS 2008). Chong and Street (2008) in a review of the clinical signs of pneumonia consider the respiratory rate to be a sensitive indicator of the presence of lower respiratory infections. The respiratory rate should therefore be assessed during the examination.

Chest wall tenderness

In a study of 965 patients, Le Gal *et al.* (2005) found that 17 per cent of the patients with a pulmonary embolus had palpable chest pain. Chest wall tenderness does not rule out significant pathology.

Expansion

A relatively small study demonstrated excellent inter- and intratester reliability when performing chest expansion measurements that was better at the xiphoid site than the axillary site. The authors of this study, however, acknowledge a lack of research into this procedure and suggest further research to establish a standard technique and large-scale data so that chest expansion measurements can be interpreted appropriately (Kalantri *et al.* 2007).

Percussion

A review of the literature on percussion, described good interobserver agreement between clinicians regarding the type of percussion note. Comparative percussion is useful in identifying a large pleural effusion but is considered to be only slightly useful in determining the presence of pneumonia (McGee 1995). This is an old review but does not appear to have been refuted in any of the more recent literature.

Auscultation of the lungs

The reliability of the stethoscope has at times been called into question. However, there is some evidence to support the hypothesis that lung sounds contain clinically important information and this supports the use of the stethoscope in clinical medicine (Murphy 2008). Although auscultation can serve to identify abnormal chest sounds, its usefulness in determining the exact cause of those sounds is limited and as with all other clinical signs, it needs to be taken in context with the history.

Crackles are due to the opening and closing of the small airways. The timing of the crackles in the respiratory cycle may serve to determine the type of disease (Talley and O'Connor 2006).

Positioning the stethoscope: There are many slight variations in different textbooks regarding where to place the stethoscope when auscultating the lungs and little hard evidence to support one over another. Recommended sites as shown in Figs 3.1 and 3.2 are based on underlying lung anatomy and the position of the scapulae.

Diaphragm or bell? Very little evidence exists regarding the benefits of using the diaphragm or the bell of the stethoscope in auscultating the lungs. Research that is available indicates that use of the diaphragm in respiratory examination is preferable to use of the bell except in the presence of chest hair (Welsby *et al.* 2003).

Can pneumonia be diagnosed on clinical examination? Considering the general consensus (but a lack of actual evidence) that a diagnosis of pneumonia should prompt early administration of antibiotics (Metlay *et al.* 1997; SIGN 2002), actually diagnosing pneumonia from clinical signs or symptoms is difficult. No combination of symptoms including respiratory rate, pulse, temperature and chest examination can reliably confirm the presence of pneumonia. This view is reiterated in a review of the evidence by Saeed and Body (2007), where it was identified that pneumonia cannot be reliably confirmed or excluded by auscultation or physical examination.

Another study of the available evidence by Woodhead *et al.* (2005) offers the following criteria to help the practitioner distinguish pneumonia from a lower respiratory tract infection:

- acute cough and one or more of the following signs/symptoms:
  - new focal chest signs
  - dyspnoea
  - tachypnoea
  - fever lasting more than 4 days.

Physicians frequently disagree on individual findings in the chest examination and if diagnostic certainty is necessary then a chest X-ray should be performed (Metlay *et al.* 1997). Further research is recommended to examine ways of improving the precision of the clinical examination.

Appropriate prescribing of antibiotics is always an issue and in a small observational cohort study of 25 general practitioners (GPs) in the Netherlands (where there is the lowest prescribing of antibiotics in Europe) the GPs frequently prescribed antibiotics for lower respiratory tract infections where there were abnormal auscultatory findings such as crackles. If antibiotics should usually only be prescribed for patients with pneumonia, the antibiotics may have been prescribed inappropriately to 86 per cent of patients and the conclusion was that GPs should consider the predictive value of clinical signs and not allow these to influence inappropriately their prescribing decisions, which should be evidence based (Hopstaken *et al.* 2006).

Terminology

There is some inconsistency in the terminology used to describe adventitious sounds. Some textbooks will still refer to crepitations or rales and rhonchi but other authors suggest adopting the use of the terms crackles (fine or coarse) and wheeze (Wilkins *et al.* 1990). For consistency and to avoid confusion it is suggested that practitioners now only use the terms 'crackles' and 'wheeze'.

 CASE STUDY

48-year-old female

Presenting complaint: Sudden onset of shortness of breath and sharp pain on inspiration.

History of presenting complaint: Recovering from total abdominal hysterectomy 10 days ago (for menorrhagia due to fibroids). Post-operative infection of wound. Shortness of breath came on suddenly 2 hours ago when getting up and has been getting steadily worse.

Medical history: Anxiety and panic attacks (but not for several years now).

Drug history: Co-codamol for post-operative pain. Lactulose for constipation (recent onset probably due to the analgesia and temporary enforced reduction in mobility). Has just completed a course of flucloxacillin for the wound infection.

Family history: Sister suffers with depression. Nil else of note.

Social History: Happily married, two teenage sons. Usually very active, enjoys outdoor sports. Non-smoker. Social drinker. Good varied diet. Works as a secondary school teacher. Job recently very stressful.

Systems review: She complains of a fast heartbeat and feels light-headed and weak. Nil else of note.
The patient appears pale and anxious and is obviously short of breath.

Test yourself

1 What are your differential diagnoses at this stage and why?
2 During the preliminary and subsequent respiratory examination which signs would help to make your diagnosis more likely?
3 Which other systems do you need to examine and why?

Answers can be found at the back of the book (p. 122).

REFLECTION ON PRACTICE

THE PATIENT WHO PRESENTED WITH A COUGH
Jane (a Nurse Practitioner) was nearing the end of morning surgery. She had to finish on time today as she had to catch a train at lunchtime. Her last patient arrived. She had triaged him on the telephone earlier that morning and from the brief history obtained then had decided the problem was likely to be a viral cough following on from a cold. She had deliberately put him in for herself because she thought this was going to be a quick consultation. She had even gone through the discussion in her head and was anticipating explaining the reason why antibiotics were not indicated and that it was likely to settle given time.

Mr Jones walked in with his wife. He looked unwell and thin. He sat down and told the story initially much as he'd presented it on the phone. He had a dry cough that had gone on for 2 weeks and wasn't settling. Jane was tempted to finish the history there, check his chest and conclude the consultation. However, something about this man's appearance made her probe a little more and take a more thorough history. It transpired that Mr Jones had been quite tired for a few months and had lost about half a stone. He showed her where his buckle was now done up two notches further in. His wife was obviously also very concerned about this. He also confessed to having some rectal bleeding, although he did have a history of haemorrhoids that had been operated on before so he assumed the bleeding was due to this. His bowels had been looser than normal lately and his appetite was not as good as it used to be. He had a family history of prostate cancer (father) and breast cancer (mother). He smoked 10 roll-ups a day. He was waiting for a right hip replacement for osteoarthritis and took paracetamol for the pain from his hip. None of this information would have been volunteered had Jane not decided to do a more thorough history.

She went on to do a full respiratory, cardiac and abdominal examination, none of which revealed anything significant. His body mass index was 20. She arranged for him to have a chest X-ray and relevant blood tests. In view of the history of weight loss and rectal bleeding Jane referred Mr Jones urgently to the rectal bleeding clinic.

The chest X-ray was normal.

Blood tests revealed a borderline anaemia and markedly raised inflammatory markers.

Further investigations revealed a malignant tumour in the descending colon.

The moral here is to allow yourself time. Remember the importance of taking a complete history, even when it seems as if the presenting complaint is relatively trivial. Examination and investigations can usually only confirm or refute an initial differential diagnosis and should never be done in isolation.

4 THE EAR, NOSE (MOUTH) AND THROAT

Zoë Rawles

Currently non-medical practitioners are often allocated the task of dealing with 'minor illness' and will increasingly find themselves faced with the task of examining the patient's ears, nose or throat. It is not a skill that is afforded a high priority in some UK medical schools (Sharma *et al.* 2006) and it seems likely that the same applies in the training of non-medics. Non-medical practitioners should seek out further training if necessary, before considering themselves competent to undertake the examination and make a diagnosis.

Perform a thorough preliminary examination first (Chapter 1), including careful palpation of the lymph nodes.

CHECKLIST

PROCEDURE	RATIONALE/POSSIBLE PATHOLOGY
EXAMINING THE EAR	
INSPECT AND PALPATE **External structure (pinna) for** • Shape and size • Deformity • Skin condition • Signs of trauma/piercing	Checking for any obvious pathology or factors that may predispose to pathology

• Signs of infection
  Erythema
  Discharge
	Otitis externa (*discharge, if present, will be thin*)
	Otitis media with perforation (*discharge will be thicker as it originates from the mucus producing cells of the middle ear*)

Rash inside ear	Ramsay Hunt syndrome type 2 (*caused by herpes zoster in the ear canal involving the geniculate ganglion and resulting in a vesicular rash together with facial palsy*)
• Inflammation	Eczema Cellulitis
• Scars/signs of previous surgery	Patients who have a history of ear surgery should usually be referred and followed-up by the specialist when there are problems

Checklist continued

• Suspicious lesions *A non-healing lesion should always be referred*	Basal cell carcinoma Squamous cell carcinoma
OTOSCOPY Hold the auriscope using the correct technique (do not use the hammer grip) (Fig. 4.1)	For safety in case of any unexpected head movement. There is less control with a hammer grip
Inspect • Ear canal: look for inflammation, debris, wax, foreign object, abnormal swelling	Otitis externa Trauma from foreign objects, e.g. hair clips, keys, cotton buds, etc Malignancy
• Tympanic membrane (TM): check for normal anatomy (Fig. 4.2) **Identify any abnormalities** • Bulging of TM/inflammation	Otitis media
• Dullness/opacity/loss of normal light reflex	Effusion
• Fluid/bubbles behind the membrane	Otitis media with effusion Glue ear
• Tympanosclerosis (*white patches seen on the tympanic membrane that may represent scarring related to chronic middle ear inflammation*)	Scarring from previous infection

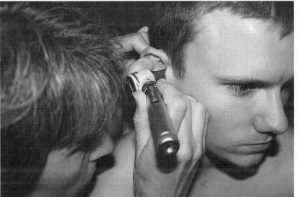

Fig. 4.1. Otoscope technique.

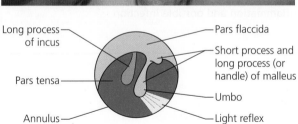

Long process of incus

Pars tensa

Annulus

Pars flaccida

Short process and long process (or handle) of malleus

Umbo

Light reflex

Fig 4.2. Diagrammatic view of a normal tympanic membrane (right ear).

Checklist continued

• Retraction of pars flaccida/tensa	Barotrauma
	Eustachian tube dysfunction
• Crusting in attic area	Wax
	Cholesteatoma (*a collection of squamous epithelium in the middle ear that may become locally invasive and destructive, causing erosion of the ossicles or mastoid bone. Because of the close proximity to the brain there is a risk of serious neurological complications*)
• Perforation	Trauma: direct/indirect
Consider the possibility of cholesteatoma where there is an unsafe perforation, i.e. on the margins or in the pars flaccida	Infection
TEST HEARING (IF PATIENT COMPLAINS OF HEARING LOSS) Using whispered voice test or Rinne and Weber (512 or 256 Hz tuning fork)	Deafness may be due to Conductive disorders Sensorineural disorders

EXAMINING THE NOSE	
INSPECT Inspect external surface and assess appearance, noting any	
• Deformity	Fracture
	Malignancy
• Inflammation	Signs indicated in the left column may be due to any of the following:
• Discharge	
• Crusting	Rhinitis
• Offensive smell	Foreign object
• Bloody/purulent discharge	Infection
	Epistaxis
• Unilateral nasal mass/ulceration	Malignancy
• Scars	Trauma/surgery
PALPATE	
• Nasal bones for tenderness	Fracture
• To determine the type of deformity, i.e. bony or cartilaginous	
• For frontal and maxillary sinus tenderness or swelling	Inflammation and possible infection

Checklist continued

EXAMINE ANTERIOR VESTIBULE View inside the anterior vestibule using a nasal speculum or auriscope **Observe**	
• Colour of mucosa	Normal nasal mucosa is reddish and moist
• Type of discharge (serous, mucoid, purulent or bloody)	Rhinitis Infection Caused by foreign object or malignancy
An offensive unilateral discharge is a 'red flag' for the presence of a foreign object when examining a child and should be managed in secondary care	
• Septum: deviation	Increases the likelihood of poor sinus drainage, breathing problems, sleep apnoea
• Scabs/bleeding points	Infection Recurrent epistaxis
• Presence of polyps/foreign objects/swelling	As a possible cause of nasal congestion, rhinitis, offensive discharge Tumour
Polyps are insensitive to touch whereas swollen turbinates will be tender	Asthma is associated with polyps
ASSESS THE SENSE OF SMELL (IF PATIENT INDICATES A PROBLEM) Refer also to the Chapter 11	
• Hyposmia/anosmia (*reduction in, or loss of, the sense of smell*)	Allergies Nasal polyps Sinusitis Upper respiratory tract infection Head trauma Space occupying lesion
• Hyperosmia (*heightened sense of smell*)	Sometimes occurs in: Migraine Cluster headaches Addison's disease

Checklist continued

EXAMINING THE MOUTH AND THROAT	
INSPECT	
The lips: externally and internally checking for	
• Angular stomatitis (*painful cracking, erythema in the angle of the lips*)	Iron, folate or vitamin B deficiency
• Inflammation, ulceration	Poorly fitting dentures
	Immunodeficiency
	Cancer
	Inflammatory bowel disease, e.g. Crohn's disease
• Nodules	May be benign or malignant
• Cyanosis	Hypoxia due to cardiovascular or respiratory disease
The teeth and gums: check for	
• Halitosis	Poor oral hygiene
	Fetor hepaticus (*sweet faecal smell, which may be a late sign of liver failure*)
	Ketoacidosis
	Cigarettes
	Alcohol
	Uraemia
	Infection
• Gingivitis: gum disease/bleeding	Vitamin C or K deficiency
	Infection
	Diabetes
	Blood dyscrasias
	Leukaemia
	Iatrogenic, e.g. due to anticoagulant therapy, phenytoin, nifedipine, oral contraception
	Pregnancy
	Dental caries
• Unexplained tooth mobility	Underlying malignancy
The tongue and the floor of the mouth: check for	
• Lingua nigra (*black tongue*)	No known cause
• Leucoplakia (*white thickened plaques or patches*)	Smoking
	Alcohol
	Poor dental hygiene
	Sepsis
	Iatrogenic
	May be pre-malignant

Checklist continued

• Hairy leucoplakia (*white corrugated or hairy patch on the side of the tongue*)	Associated with HIV and/or immunosuppression
• Glossitis (*smooth and sometimes erythematous tongue*)	Iron, folate or vitamin B deficiency
• Swelling of sublingual/submandibular glands	Occasionally stones will form in the sublingual glands although the majority form in the submandibular glands
The mouth (buccal area and space between cheek and gums): check for	
• Ulcers	Aphthous ulcers: cause usually not obvious but may be due to:
	Crohn's disease
	Coeliac disease
	HIV infection
	Ulcers persisting for longer than 3 weeks may be a sign of malignancy
• Lumps/overgrowth of tissue	**Malignancy**
• Creamy white patches (thrush) and/or erythema	Immunosuppression
	Following use of systemic antibiotics
	Diabetes
	Iron deficiency
	Lichen planus (*self-limiting itchy rash that may affect the mouth, skin, nails and hair*)
	Erythema multiformae (*a skin condition that varies from mild self-limiting disease to serious and potentially fatal which also affects mucous membranes*)
	Oral cancer
The oropharynx: check	
• Uvula: swelling, deviation	Tonsillar abscess
	Cranial nerve IX palsy
• Soft palate: asymmetry or abnormality	Quinsy (*peritonsillar abscess*)
	Malignancy
• Tonsils for inflammation, swelling, ulceration, exudate	Tonsillitis
	Glandular Fever
Tonsillar exudate associated with tender anterior cervical lymph nodes, absence of a cough and history of fever make up the **Centor criteria**. *When three or four of these criteria occur together, it is more likely to indicate infection with Group A beta-haemolytic Streptococcus (GABHS)*	
PALPATE (WEARING GLOVES) If necessary, inside the mouth and under the tongue for any abnormal swellings	To determine the characteristics of the swelling

THE EVIDENCE

Otoscopy

This can only be performed accurately and safely by using the correct technique. The Rotherham Ear Care Centre is a leading authority on ear care in the UK and the correct technique for using the otoscope is described in their guidelines (Harkin 2008) and demonstrated in Fig 4.1.

Otitis media

This is the term used to describe middle ear inflammation – occurring acutely or chronically, with or without symptoms. It is classified clinically as acute otitis media (AOM) and otitis media with effusion (OME), but it is not always easy to distinguish between the two (Hoberman and Paradise 2000). The former is usually symptomatic and may present with systemic illness, whereas the latter is often asymptomatic. More research is needed to determine the link between language delay and/or behavioural problems with persistent OME. A review of the available evidence concludes that children with OME should not be treated with antibiotics (Scottish Intercollegiate Guidelines Network 2003).

Whispered voice test

A systematic review of studies of test accuracy concluded that the whispered voice test is an accurate and simple test for detecting hearing impairment (Pirozzo *et al.* 2003). The test sensitivity was however much lower for children, and in the absence of any clear evidence to the contrary, they should always be referred for audiometry.

Rinne and Weber tests (tuning fork tests)

The Rinne test is positive when air conduction is louder than bone conduction but although it will reliably test a conduction defect, it is no substitute for pure audiometry (Tidy 2008).

The Weber test can be used to demonstrate a conductive or a sensorineural hearing loss but it is less accurate (McGee 2001). Tuning fork tests should always follow hearing tests as they cannot distinguish normal hearing from bilateral sensorineural loss.

A review of 24 studies on the accuracy of hearing tests (Bagai *et al.* 2006) concluded that elderly people who perceived the whispered voice test did not require further testing but those who could not required audiometry. On the basis of their findings the authors also advised against the use of Rinne and Weber tests for general screening.

Mouth cancer

In 2004 there were 7697 cases of mouth cancer in the UK and late detection has a significant effect on mortality rates. One person will die every 3 hours in the UK from mouth cancer (Mouth Cancer Foundation 2008) so attention to the history and careful examination is vital.

Sore throat

This is a self-limiting condition and will resolve in 85 per cent of patients within 1 week whether or not it is due to a streptococcal infection. (Del Mar *et al.* 2004). Tonsillar exudate alone does not mean that a prescription for antibiotics should be inevitable and the Centor criteria (Centor *et al.* 1981), as outlined in the checklist, are still used as a tool to determine the need for antimicrobial treatment

(MeReC 2006). Current advice is against the routine use of antibiotics in upper respiratory infections in people who are otherwise well and evidence indicates that more than 4000 people would need to be given antibiotics to prevent one case of quinsy (MeReC 2008).

REFLECTION ON PRACTICE

THE PATIENT WITH A SORE THROAT

Mrs Hughes was a 50-year-old lady, a known alcoholic and heavy smoker: a typical 'heart sink' patient. She was underweight and looked unwell. She was a frequent attendee, who had sometimes been quite disruptive, turning up and demanding to be seen without an appointment. The receptionists and doctors were well used to her and felt they had reached the 'end of the road' with her in terms of what they could do.

She presented on one occasion with a severe sore throat, worse on the left side that had gone on for a few weeks and showed no signs of settling. Unfortunately when she came in her breath smelt of alcohol and she was a little confused. The General Practitioner (GP) examined her throat and could see no evidence of infection so he suggested she try ibuprofen and paracetamol.

Two weeks later she attended again, this time quite sober. She was trying very hard to give up the alcohol and had managed to stay 'dry' for 5 days now. She was again examined and although the GP could still see no evidence of infection she was given a course of penicillin.

Three weeks later she attended again and this time was again slightly the worse for wear after drinking quite heavily in the morning and taking co-codamol for her painful throat. This time she was given a course of ciproxin.

Three weeks later she came in and the GP asked the Nurse Practitioner to see her as he was inundated with several 'fit-ins'. The nurse was helping out for the day and was unfamiliar with Mrs Hughes' history. She complained of a persisting painful throat with severe constant pain, not relieved with co-codamol or ibuprofen. Her symptoms had now gone on for nearly 3 months and were getting worse. She could no longer swallow any solid food and was now also having problems swallowing fluids. She wore a scarf around her neck and held her throat as if trying to reduce the pain. She was unable to sleep because of it.

The practitioner could not see anything in her mouth or throat but in view of the symptoms, she made an urgent referral to ear nose and throat (ENT) and prescribed stronger analgesia.

Ten days later Mrs Hughes came into reception in a very distressed state, explaining angrily that she had just been diagnosed with throat cancer and demanding to know why it had taken a nurse to discover this. The ENT consultant told her she should have been referred weeks ago and she was going to file a complaint.

This story is not meant to be a criticism of doctors or to suggest that Nurse Practitioners are in some way better. Obviously at this stage the doctor would also have referred Mrs Hughes, it just happened that it was the nurse she saw. It is however a true story and does demonstrate how easy it is to stop listening to the 'heart sink' patient who presents on multiple occasions and appears beyond help.

(Significant in Mrs Hughes history was the alcohol abuse and cigarette smoking, which both increase the risk of throat cancer. It was also the slowly increasing and constant nature of the pain that was suggestive of a sinister cause.)

CASE STUDY

36-year-old male

Presenting complaint: Persistent discharge from right ear. Feeling of heaviness and discomfort on the same side. Reduced hearing on the same side also.

History of presenting complaint: Symptoms have persisted for 3–4 weeks now.

Medical history: Recurrent ear infections. Type 1 diabetes (well controlled).

continued ➤

CASE STUDY *continued*

Drug history: Insulin. Aspirin. Paracetamol for ear ache as necessary.

Family history: Nil relevant.

Social history: Computer analyst. Happily married with two children. Lives in own home. No financial problems. Smokes five a day. Drinks approximately 20 units alcohol throughout the week. Eats a healthy diet. Enjoys exercise such as swimming and cycling.

Systems review: Nil relevant.

Preliminary examination

Temperature: 37.2°C.
Pulse 78 beats per minute.
Swollen and tender auricular and cervical lymph nodes on the right side.
Mouth and throat: NAD (no abnormality detected).
All else normal.

Test yourself

1 You notice an offensive odour from the ear. When you examine the right ear there is some debris and the ear canal is inflamed. Consider the history and explain why it is important to do an ear swab for this patient?

2 Despite the debris you are able to visualize the tympanic membrane. There is a perforation in the attic area (pars flaccida). What type of perforation is this?

3 What are your differential diagnoses?

4 Which other procedure could be done as part of the examination?

5 Which factors in the history may predispose to recurrent ear infections?

Answers are to be found at the back of the book (p. 122).

5

THE ABDOMEN

Trudy Alexander

The following list encompasses the main techniques for examination of the abdomen. It is however only necessary to perform those techniques that are indicated by the patient's history and the rest of the examination. For instance, it is unnecessary to check for Murphy's sign if there is no upper abdominal pain, and if the liver is normal on palpation and percussion it would be fruitless to check for liver bruits.

An integrated examination may be necessary when the working differential diagnosis includes pathology originating in other systems. It may for example be necessary to examine the cardiovascular system when the presenting complaint is epigastric pain.

Perform a thorough preliminary examination first. Of particular significance are brittleness and spooning of the fingernails, finger clubbing, pale mucous membranes, jaundice, palmar erythema, liver flap, enlarged clavicular lymph nodes, rashes and an enlarged thyroid gland.

CHECKLIST	
PROCEDURE	**RATIONALE/POSSIBLE PATHOLOGY**
INSPECT • The mouth and throat: refer to Chapter 4	
ABDOMEN **Observe for** • Signs of pain	Lying still limits pain from peritoneal irritation A person with intestinal or renal colic may keep changing position in an effort to relieve the pain
• Generalized or localized distension/swelling Check contour of abdomen In conjunction with abdominal auscultation may be useful in the diagnosis of acute small bowel obstruction	Fat: obesity may be associated with diseases such as cholecystitis Fluid: bulging flanks may be due to ascites. Refer to ascites section further down this list Flatus Faeces Fetus Hernia Enlarged liver, spleen or gall bladder Tumour
• Visible peristalsis	Obstruction

Checklist continued

• Pulsation of the aorta (expansile impulse)	**Abdominal Aortic aneurysm**
• Absence of movement	Peritonitis
• Scaphoid abdomen	Malnourished and underweight
	Anorexia
	Carcinoma
	Inflammatory bowel disease (Fig. 5.1)
• Striae	Rapid weight gain such as during pregnancy
	Obesity
	Cushing's syndrome
	Long-term use of cortisone
• Caput medusae (*engorged abdominal veins radiating from the umbilicus*)	Sign of portal hypertension which may be due to cirrhosis of the liver
• Spider naevi (*superficial dilated blood vessels with central red spot resembling a spider. Up to 1 cm in diameter and normally above the waist*)	Chronic liver disease. Significance increased if five or more
• Scars	Operations or injuries. May be associated with adhesions
• Jaundice	Pre-hepatic: gallstones, carcinoma of the pancreas and drugs/poisons
	Hepatic: hepatitis, cirrhosis
	Post hepatic: excess haemolysis of red blood cells

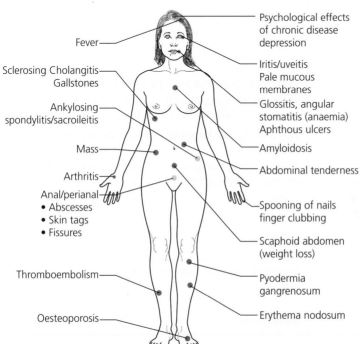

Fig. 5.1. Signs associated with inflammatory bowel disease.

Checklist continued

• Cullen's sign (peri-umbilical ecchymosis) Grey Turner's sign (ecchymosis of the flanks)	Signs of retroperitoneal haemorrhage seen in intra-abdominal catastrophes such as: Acute haemorrhagic pancreatitis Ruptured ectopic pregnancy Bilateral salpingitis Intestinal strangulation
• Collateral venous circulation	Portal hypertension Obstruction of inferior or superior vena cava
Auscultate (Fig. 5.2) For bruits over the	
• Aorta Renal arteries Iliac arteries	Stenosis Aneurysm
• **The liver**	Hepatoma
• For bowel sounds **abdominal auscultation** is useful in acute abdominal pain	
Hypoactive	Paralytic ileus Peritonitis (known as the still silent abdomen)
Hyperactive	Diarrhoea Constipation Early small bowel obstruction

49

50

Fig. 5.2. Auscultation sites for abdominal bruits.

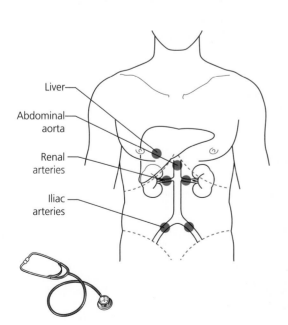

Liver

Abdominal aorta

Renal arteries

Iliac arteries

Checklist continued

Percuss

• Over the four abdominal quadrants	
To identify and outline any masses	Cysts, tumours, faeces, abscess
To gauge the severity of tenderness prior to palpation	Inflammation
	Infection
	In peritonitis light percussion may be painful
• To identify suspected **ascites**:	Liver disease
	Portal vein obstruction
Test for shifting dullness	Malnutrition
Gaseous bowel floats on top of fluid, which is why the flanks are dull when the patient is supine. When the patient turns the fluid migrates and the dull note changes position	Malignancy
	Infection
	Nephrotic syndrome
	Constrictive pericarditis
Test for a positive fluid wave	Heart failure
• The **liver**	Cirrhosis
For hepatomegaly	Infections such as hepatitis
Identify the upper and lower borders of the liver in the mid-clavicular line (Fig. 5.3)	Congestion such as in cardiac failure
	Malignancy
	Inflammation
• Across the area known as **Traube's space** (Fig. 5.3)	Infectious, neoplastic and congestive disorders such as:
	Leukaemia
Normally the spleen will not be detected in this area unless enlarged	Lymphoma

(50) (49) (48)

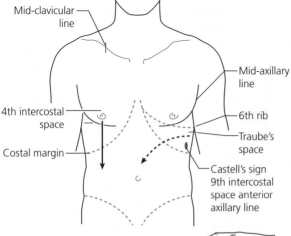

Mid-clavicular line

Mid-axillary line

4th intercostal space

6th rib

Traube's space

Costal margin

Castell's sign 9th intercostal space anterior axillary line

Liver percussion

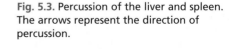
Percussion across Traube's space

Percussion for Castell's sign

Fig. 5.3. Percussion of the liver and spleen. The arrows represent the direction of percussion.

Checklist continued

49 • In the lowest left intercostal space of the anterior axillary line during expiration and inspiration. The percussion note changes from resonant on expiration to dull on inspiration in splenomegaly **Castell's sign** (Fig. 5.3). *Useful if an enlarged spleen is suspected but it is not palpable*	Infectious mononucleosis Malaria Thalassaemia Cirrhosis of the liver
• The costophrenic angle in order to elicit tenderness	Pyelonephritis Renal abscess Calculus Infarction
47 **Palpate (abdominal palpation)** • Lightly and then more deeply in all four quadrants	
To localize any tender or painful areas and to determine the severity. To check for guarding	Localized or generalized peritonitis Inflammation of any underlying structure
To locate any palpable masses	Carcinoma, abscess, cyst, faecal impaction
47 • For rebound tenderness (**abdominal palpation**)	Localized or generalized peritonitis
• For an expansile impulse of the aorta	In a non-obese patient it is sometimes possible to palpate an **abdominal aortic aneurysm** 50
49 • The **liver** edge: (Fig. 5.4) To determine whether the liver is enlarged	Cirrhosis Infections such as hepatitis
Liver size should be assessed in conjunction with liver percussion. A palpable liver is not always enlarged or diseased but the likelihood of hepatomegaly is increased	Congestion such as in cardiac failure Malignancy Inflammation
To determine the characteristics of the liver edge:	
Firm	Cirrhosis
Nodular	Cirrhosis and malignancy. Nodules are generally larger in malignancy
Tender	Infection or swelling
Pulsatile	Tricuspid valve disease or constrictive pericarditis
51 • For **Murphy's sign** in the mid-clavicular line of the right costal margin. Tenderness is elicited on inspiration	Specific for acute cholecystitis

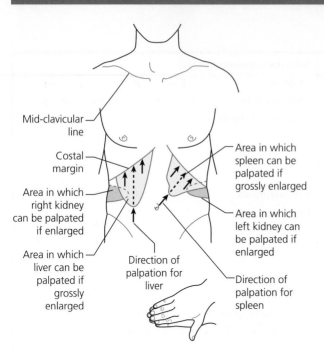

Fig. 5.4. Palpation for enlarged abdominal organs. The arrows represent the direction of palpation.

Mid-clavicular line

Costal margin

Area in which right kidney can be palpated if enlarged

Area in which liver can be palpated if grossly enlarged

Direction of palpation for liver

Area in which spleen can be palpated if grossly enlarged

Area in which left kidney can be palpated if enlarged

Direction of palpation for spleen

Checklist continued

• **The spleen** (Fig. 5.4) To detect an enlarged spleen in conjunction with percussion. Usually only palpable when grossly enlarged *Omit if there is risk of rupture such as in infectious mononucleosis*	Infectious, neoplastic and congestive disorders such as: Leukaemia Lymphoma Infectious mononucleosis Malaria Thalassaemia Cirrhosis of the liver
• **The kidneys** (Fig. 5.3) *May be felt in a thin patient but this does not always indicate significant pathology*	Polycystic kidney disease Hydronephrosis Carcinoma
• For an enlarged uterus in a female Refer to Chapter 6 for pelvic examination	Pregnancy Carcinoma Fibroids Hydatidiform mole
• For hernias Ask the patient to cough and check for an expansile impulse. Check the scrotum in a male and repeat with the patient standing if necessary *If a hernia cannot be reduced strangulation may occur*	Inguinal Femoral Incisional Paraumbilical Epigastric

Checklist continued

• For enlarged inguinal lymph nodes	Localized infection
	Generalized diseases such as lymphoma or carcinoma
• For an enlarged urinary bladder in conjunction with percussion	Urinary retention due to obstruction or neurological disorders
	Tumours
RECTAL EXAMINATION Carry out if necessary	
• Inspect the sacrococcygeal anal and perianal area for abnormalities	Fissures, fistulas and skin infections may be associated with chronic conditions such as Crohn's disease (inflammatory bowel disease) (Fig 5.1 on p 42).
	Warts, fungal skin infections, haemorrhoids, skin tags, abscesses, pilonidal cysts or rectal prolapse
• Perform a **digital rectal examination** Check for sphincter, rectal and prostate abnormalities such as:	
Laxity of the anal sphincter	Neurological lesion
Tightness	Scarring
Spasticity	Fissure, inflammation or anxiety
A lump or mass	Distal tumour, enlarged prostate
Tender areas	Inflammatory bowel disease, infection, haemorrhoids
Refer to Chapter 6 for prostate abnormalities	
Check the glove for blood and mucous	Distal tumours
	Diverticulitis
	Inflammatory bowel disease
	Haemorrhoids

48

THE EVIDENCE

Abdominal palpation

Experience appears to be a factor in clinical examination of the abdomen. Pines *et al.* (2005) compared the findings between attending and resident physicians in the USA, for tenderness, guarding, masses and distension in 122 patients. There was almost perfect agreement for masses but only moderate agreement for tenderness, guarding and distension.

There are conflicting studies regarding rebound tenderness. Liddington and Thomson (1991) in a study involving 142 patients with abdominal pain and tenderness found it to be of no predictive value. In contrast with this, Alshehri *et al.* (1995), who studied 123 patients with a diagnosis of acute appendicitis, found it to be a highly sensitive test with a good negative predictive value. It did not however have good specificity and did not have a good positive predictive value. Golledge *et al.* (1996) in a study of 100 patients with right iliac fossa pain found the converse to be true, with rebound tenderness having a good positive predictive value.

Acute appendicitis is historically difficult to diagnose, with many patients undergoing unnecessary surgery while others suffer adverse consequences when they are misdiagnosed and do not have surgery. Andersson *et al.* (2000) studied 496 patients and considered the variables that influenced the surgeons' decision to operate. It was discovered that the surgeons placed too strong an emphasis on pain and tenderness, and paid less attention to the duration of symptoms and objective signs of inflammation.

Another study by Graff *et al.* (2000) looked at 1026 patients who had an appendicectomy and 1118 patients who presented with abdominal pain. They found that some patients with appendicitis have few clinical findings whereas some patients without appendicitis have clinical findings similar to those of patients with appendicitis and this can lead to diagnostic errors. Adverse events were related to false-negative decisions.

It is clear that larger, more up-to-date and reliable studies are needed to inform the practitioners' decision-making regarding abdominal examination. From the information available however it appears that both patient and examiner variables affect findings and that findings must be considered within the context of a full history and other signs. Where there is doubt a second opinion should be sought or the patient referred. A period of hospital observation may help to clarify the diagnosis.

The **rebound test** is painful and should be used with discretion. In patients where there is already tenderness, guarding and/or signs of inflammation such as pyrexia and vomiting, it may serve no useful purpose as the examiner should have enough information to make a decision. Establishing a diagnosis for acute abdominal pain is however often elusive and a negative rebound test may be a useful adjunct in the armoury of diagnostic tools.

Digital rectal examination

Ang *et al.* (2008) in a study involving 1069 patients referred by General Practitioners (GPs), found that digital rectal examination (DRE) for palpable rectal tumours was inaccurate in terms of both positive and negative predictive values. In addition, less than 10 per cent of colorectal cancers occur within reach of the examining finger (United States Preventative Services Task Force 2003).

Digital rectal examination is an uncomfortable and often embarrassing procedure for the patient and if a rectal tumour is suspected the patient will be referred urgently for further investigation regardless of DRE results. The examiner should therefore use their discretion regarding whether rectal examination would be useful for their patient. In certain circumstances it may be justified, especially in areas where there are longer consultant waiting times and a positive finding should afford the patient some priority on the waiting list.

The spleen

Traube's space

Several small studies have compared different methods of palpation and percussion with ultrasound. Tamayo *et al.* (1993) compared three methods of palpation and three methods of percussion with ultrasound using eight examiners and 27 patients. All tests were relatively insensitive but specific. Results varied according to the examiner and this was not related to experience. Combining tests increased diagnostic accuracy. Barkun *et al.* (1989) looked at the influence of meals and obesity on Traube's space percussion and found that accuracy was increased by performing the examination 2 hours after a meal and in non-obese patients. The method did not obviate the need for further diagnostic testing. Barkun *et al.* (1991) compared five methods of percussion and palpation with ultrasound. No method of palpation was found to be superior and palpation was most accurate in lean patients. The optimal examination was percussion of Traube's space, followed by palpation if percussion was dull. Dubey *et al.* (2000) compared palpation and percussion of Traube's space (Barkun's method) with ultrasound. The accuracy improved when both methods were combined.

Castell's sign

A 1993 systematic review found that Castell's sign, if combined with other clinical findings, was the most sensitive manoeuvre to detect splenomegaly (Grover *et al.* 1993). The probability of the presence of splenomegaly based upon the history and other signs should however be 70 per cent. It was found to be superior to palpation unless the spleen is grossly enlarged. The spleen may then be palpated below the costal margin. It is not sufficiently sensitive to rule an enlarged spleen in or out (Grover *et al.* 1993). A further study involving 80 patients compared two methods of palpation and three of percussion (Chongtham *et al.* 1997a). The findings suggested that palpatory methods such as Middleton's manoeuvre and supine palpation could be used for diagnosing splenomegaly in non-obese patients. In this later study Castell's sign was highly sensitive but had poor specificity.

Overall the studies are old, small and inconclusive. There does however appear to be a consensus that accuracy is improved by combining both palpation and percussion. It may also be wise to examine the patient at least 2 hours after a meal where practical. Findings are often inaccurate in terms of both positive and negative predictability, especially in obese patients. If an enlarged spleen is not found but is suspected further investigations are warranted.

The liver

Joshi *et al.* (2004) studied three doctors using palpation and percussion to diagnose hepatomegaly in 180 patients and compared the results with ultrasound findings. There was modest agreement but the study suggested that palpation and percussion were not sufficiently accurate to confirm or exclude hepatomegaly. Other factors in the history and examination need to be considered. This supported the findings of earlier less rigorous studies.

A less robust study that compared palpation, light percussion and auscultatory percussion for detecting the liver below the costal margin in 45 normal subjects and 20 patients reported results indicating that all methods were valuable for detecting liver disease (Gilbert 1994).

An analysis of the evidence in 'The rational clinical examination' (Naylor 1994), suggests that liver examination is only useful where the history and other physical signs are suggestive of a hepatobiliary complaint. It is stated that both palpation and percussion are useful in assessing liver size and that palpation of the liver edge is useful if there are signs of liver disease. Detection of a palpable liver seems to be easier when the consistency of the liver is firm. A palpable liver edge may not indicate hepatomegaly but it increases the likelihood of it.

Auscultation of the liver for bruits appears to have a limited role in routine examination when the liver is found to be enlarged.

Naylor (1994) made some useful recommendations regarding examination of the liver.

- Where palpation and percussion are normal and there is a low probability of liver disease, hepatomegaly is unlikely.
- Where there is a low probability of disease but the liver edge is palpable and the liver span is less than 12–13 cm then hepatomegaly is unlikely.

- Where there is high probability of disease and the liver edge cannot be palpated it may be possible to measure span by percussion alone. Results however vary according to whether percussion is light, moderate or heavy.
- If the liver edge is palpable and there is hepatomegaly plus other signs of liver disease then the quality of the liver edge should be assessed.

In the absence of more up-to-date studies, it is recommended that when further investigations cannot be easily accessed, the patient with suspected liver disease should be referred regardless of examination results.

Ascites

Chongtham *et al.* (1997b, 1998) carried out two studies each involving 66 patients with suspected ascites. Auscultatory percussion, the puddle sign, flank dullness, the fluid wave sign and ultrasound were compared. Auscultatory percussion was the most sensitive but it was not highly specific. The fluid wave sign was poorly sensitive but the most specific. None of the manoeuvres were found to be reliable enough to predict positively or negatively ascites.

A systematic review by Williams and Simel (1992) also found that no single sign is both sensitive and specific, but they did comment that the best predictors for ascites were a positive fluid wave and shifting dullness, while the absence of bulging flanks, flank dullness and shifting dullness were useful negative predictors.

On the basis of current available evidence it is recommended that a combination of procedures to elicit the signs described by Williams and Simel (1992) may be useful. Where the history is suggestive of significant disease, further investigations should be carried out regardless of results.

Abdominal aortic aneurysm

The pooled data from studies indicate that abdominal palpation directed at measuring aortic width could not exclude abdominal aortic aneurysm (AAA) especially if rupture is a possibility, but it was moderately sensitive enough to pick up an AAA large enough to be referred for surgery. Sensitivity is reduced in obesity (Lederle and Simel 1999). This is supported by a study involving 200 patients conducted by Fink *et al.* (2000). Another study involving 4171 men who were examined for AAA by GPs found that palpation for an aortic aneurysm was clinically worthwhile even though not all aneurysms are detected (Zuhrie *et al.* 1999). Since AAAs may remain asymptomatic until they rupture the diagnosis is important. Lederle and Simel (1999) suggest that patients with first-degree relatives who have had an AAA and men over 65 should have ultrasound screening.

Abdominal auscultation

Eskelinen *et al.* (1994) examined the accuracy of the clinical diagnosis of acute small bowel obstruction in 1333 patients with acute abdominal pain. The most valuable clinical signs were **abdominal distension** and abnormal bowel sounds. This in conjunction with previous abdominal surgery and type of abdominal pain were strong indicators.

A study involving eight patients and four healthy volunteers analysed the assessment of recorded intestinal sounds by 100 physicians (Gade *et al.* 1998). Agreement was acceptable in normal subjects and those with intestinal obstruction but there was disagreement for peritonitis. It was concluded that auscultation is useful in patients with acute abdominal pain.

Current research supports the inclusion of auscultation for bowel sounds in the abdominal examination of patients with acute abdominal pain particularly where small bowel obstruction is suspected. Additional information may be obtained which may aid diagnosis.

Murphy's sign

Urbano and Carroll (2000) in a review of Murphy's sign found that there were relatively few studies evaluating its accuracy but concluded that it is a useful diagnostic tool when cholecystitis is suspected. They do however state that practitioners must also consider laboratory and imaging studies and evaluate each case individually.

If there is a high index of suspicion following the history and examination then further investigation may need to be carried out. However even 'gold standard' tests for specific pathologies can give false-negative or false-positive results. Investigations can reveal pathology that may or may not be significant. Gallstones for instance are often found but their presence does not always cause symptoms. As always, examination findings and investigation results must be considered within the context of the history.

REFLECTION ON PRACTICE

RECORD KEEPING AND VIGILANCE
Alison was a 20-year-old woman who had been seen by her local practitioner several times in the last year. She had been diagnosed with gastroenteritis each time. At this visit Alison's mother came with her. There was a sense of urgency in the mother's voice and Alison looked thin and pale. She complained of intermittent diarrhoea that had been going on for 9 months. Each episode of diarrhoea was lasting for longer and was accompanied by cramp-like abdominal pain. She was feeling weak and unwell. The records did not contain any details of the history or examination for previous consultations. The entries simply contained the diagnoses of gastroenteritis. It was difficult therefore to make any comparison.

A preliminary examination and full abdominal examination were carried out. Alison was underweight with a body mass index of 17. There were some small painful fissures in the corners of her mouth (angular stomatitis) and on inspection the abdomen was scaphoid in appearance due to weight loss. On deep palpation Alison complained of tenderness particularly in the right iliac fossa.

Blood tests were carried out and Alison was referred urgently for gastrointestinal investigations. The blood tests revealed anaemia, an elevated white cell count and elevated erythrocyte sedimentation rate. Gastrointestinal investigations demonstrated that Alison was suffering from inflammatory bowel disease affecting mainly the small intestine. She is now being treated for Crohn's disease and is currently well.

This story demonstrates the importance of record-keeping and vigilance. Clinical signs are not always apparent initially. If careful records are kept then subsequent examiners can compare findings and may be alerted earlier to possible significant pathology. In this case an earlier referral based upon Alison's history may have prevented the deterioration in her condition. Many negligence cases are based upon inadequate record-keeping and delayed diagnosis.

CASE STUDY

28-year-old female

Presenting complaint: Abdominal discomfort and nausea for 5 days.

Recurrent sore throat, cough, intermittent fever, swollen lymph nodes and general tiredness for the last 6 months.

Past medical history: Nil of note.

Medication: Paracetamol for frequent headaches.

Family history: Mother suffers from hypertension and father from rheumatoid arthritis.

All other family members alive and well.

Ethnic origin of father is white Caucasian and ethnic origin of mother is black African.

Social history: Works as a vet for large animals and travels to Africa as part of her work. Returned from her last trip 3 weeks ago.

Non-smoker.

Drinks 15–25 units of wine per week.

Lives alone but has a boyfriend who lives in Africa.

Systems review: Irregular menstruation for the last 6 months. Last menstruation was 3 months ago.

Nil of note otherwise.

Test yourself

1 What are your differential diagnoses at this stage?
2 On examination you note that there is yellowing of the sclera and evidence of weight loss. What other physical signs would you look for?
3 What other factors do you need to consider?

Answers can be found at the back of the book (p. 122).

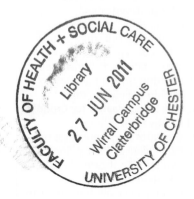

6 THE GENITOURINARY SYSTEM

Beth Griffiths

Key points for genitourinary examination

Last menstrual period

The date of the last menstrual period should be noted and pregnancy considered before examination.

Distress

Patients may find this examination very traumatic especially if there is a history of sexual abuse or rape and this should be explored prior to the examination.

Examine

Patients often request to be examined by a same-sex clinician and this should be respected. Consider whether the examination is really necessary. Women who have an imperforate hymen and need a full gynaecological examination should be examined by a specialist.

Chaperones

All patients should be offered a chaperone and if refused this should be documented. The presence of a chaperone in subsequent examinations should be mandatory in patients who react abnormally to the examination. The documentation should reflect this.

Consent

It is particularly important in this examination to pay careful attention to the consent procedure. Does the patient have the ability to consent to this examination? Has consent been given freely? Do they understand the reasons for the examination? No one else has the right to consent on behalf of another competent adult (Department of Health 2001)

Perform a preliminary examination first. Particular attention should be paid to oral mucosa and the skin for clues of systemic illness such as lichen planus and psoriasis. Associated symptoms such as arthritis and inflammation of the eyes can indicate Reiter's syndrome or Behçet's disease. Abnormal hair distribution and hirsutism may also be significant findings.

Refer to Chapter 5 before this examination as an abdominal examination should precede any genitourinary assessment.

Examination of the kidneys, bladder and hernias are covered in the Chapter 5.

The rectovaginal examination has been omitted from the text as it is not routinely carried out except by specialist clinicians.

CHECKLIST

PROCEDURE	RATIONALE/POSSIBLE PATHOLOGY
MALE Patient may be lying or standing **Inspection of the penis for**	
• Contour	Unusual curvatures: Peyronie's disease (penile fibromatosis, usually only seen when penis is erect)
	Rarely, a priapism may be present (prolonged penile erection: this can be idiopathic but can also occur in patients with leukaemia or sickle cell anaemia, and neurological conditions)
• State of foreskin	Phimosis (can't retract foreskin)
	Paraphimosis (can't replace retracted foreskin)
	Previous circumcision
• Site of urethral meatus	Hypospadias (the meatus is ventral and more proximal than normal)
	Epispadias (the meatus is dorsal)
	Both of these conditions are congenital but can be an indication of underlying abnormalities such as undescended testicles, chromosomal disorders or Klinfelter's syndrome
• Evidence of infection	Balanitis (inflammation of the glans penis)
	Warts
	Sebaceous cysts
	Sexually transmitted infections
• Any swellings Papules (*small raised lumps/lesions above the skin, <5 mm*)	Hair follicles
	Sebaceous glands
Nodules (*same as papule but larger <10 mm*)	Tyson's glands ('*pearly papules, skin coloured around the circumference of the glans' crown, often mistaken for warts, but are non-infectious*)
	Molluscum contagiosum
	Genital warts
	Lichen planus
	Psoriasis
	Dermatitis
	Balanitis
	Can be due to poor hygiene
Plaques (*palpable lesions >10 mm in diameter that are elevated above the skin surface*)	Psoriasis
	Molluscum contagiosum (*larger lesions seen in acquired immunodeficiency syndrome (AIDS) patients*)
	Erythroplasia of Queyrat (*solitary or multiple erythematous plaques, can be precancerous*)
Macules (*completely flat, change in skin colour or texture*)	Lichen sclerosus/balanitis xerotica obliterans can degenerate into penile cancer

Checklist continued

• Ulceration	
Single ulcer	Primary syphilis
	Chancroid lymphogranuloma (*chlamydial infection which infects squamocolumnar epithelial cells*)
	Penile carcinoma
Multiple ulcers	Secondary syphilis
	Herpes simplex/zoster
	Penile carcinoma
Chronic ulceration	Pemphigus vulgaris (*a rare, relapsing autoimmune disease causing blistering of the skin and mucous membranes, e.g. mouth, nose, throat and genitals*)
	Behçet's disease (*an autoimmune disorder causing inflammation, especially of the small blood vessels – vasculitis*)
	Reiter's syndrome (autoimmune condition that develops in response to an infection in another part of the body, usually affecting joints, eyes and urethra)
• Urethral discharge	Is uncommon without infection
The presence of skin lesions or discharge may require sampling of the area via swabs or biopsy	
• Parasites	Pediculosis (lice)
	Pthirus pubis (crab louse)
• Scrotum for skin abnormalities	Fungal infections
	Sebaceous cysts
	Sexually transmitted infections
	Unusual thickening of the scrotal sac may be caused by generalized fluid retention as in cardiac, hepatic or renal disease
Palpate the	
• Penis: *almost all of the examination of the penis is carried out by inspection; palpation is only indicated when an abnormality is present. Ask patient to withdraw foreskin and then replace after examination*	
• Scrotum for	
Presence of the testes	Undescended testicles
Abnormal painful swelling	Acute epididymitis
	Orchitis
	Torsion of the spermatic cord
	Strangulated inguinal hernia
Non-tender swellings (Fig. 6.1)	Indirect inguinal hernias

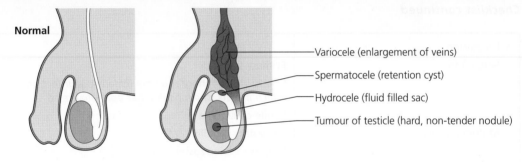

Normal

Variocele (enlargement of veins)

Spermatocele (retention cyst)

Hydrocele (fluid filled sac)

Tumour of testicle (hard, non-tender nodule)

Fig. 6.1. Genitourinary examination.

Checklist continued

Transilluminate testing will help to differentiate between fluid-filled swellings or solid tissue. Fluid-filled swellings transmit light (e.g. hydrocele and spermatocele) whereas solid masses do not	Sebaceous cysts are common in the superficial skin of the scrotum Varicocele (*abnormal enlargement of the veins in the scrotum*) (*negative to transillumination*) Spermatocele (*benign retention cyst*) Hydrocele (*a fluid collection within the tunica vaginalis of the scrotum or along the spermatic cord*)
• Testicles *Should be smooth, rubbery and free of nodules, sensitive but not tender*	Abnormalities may indicate infection or the presence of a cyst or **tumour**. Testicular cancer is usually a hard non-tender nodule. If suspected check for **gynaecomastia** Soft, small testicles may indicate cirrhosis or hypogonadism
If absent check along their line of descent.	Cryptorchidism (undescended testicle)
• Spermatic cord	Thickening of the vas deferens may be due to chronic infection A varicocele may also be felt along the length of the cord (only when standing) (Fig 6.1)
FEMALE **Inspect the** • Vulva for Excoriation	Dermatitis and *Candida* infection can cause irritation Lichen sclerosus (can be a premalignant condition) Psoriasis Paget's disease (*chronic eczema-like rash of the skin around the anogenital regions, 25 per cent associated with underlying cancer*)
Varicosities/oedema	Varicosities can occur in the labia Oedema is common in pregnancy

Checklist continued

Nodular or papular lesions	Molluscum contagiosum
	Genital warts
	Secondary syphilis
	Sebaceous cysts are commonly found in the labial area. Fordyce's spots inside the labia minora are normal (*yellow/white papules*)
Swellings	May be due to prolapse which is visible at introitus (cystocele, rectocele or procedentia)
	A urethral caruncle appears as a red fleshy lesion at the urethral meatus
Discharge	Abnormal vaginal or urethral discharges are representative of infection.
Single ulcerated lesions	Primary syphilis,
	Vulval carcinoma
	Chancroid lymphogranuloma (*chlamydial infection which infects squamocolumnar epithelial cells*)
Multiple lesions	Herpetic infection
	Secondary syphilis
Chronic ulceration	Pemphigus vulgaris (*a rare, relapsing autoimmune disease causing blistering of the skin and mucous membranes, e.g. mouth, nose, throat and genitals*)
	Behçet's disease (*an autoimmune disorder causing inflammation, especially of the small blood vessels – vasculitis*)
	Reiter's syndrome (*autoimmune condition that develops in response to an infection in another part of the body, usually affecting joints, eyes and urethra*)
Bruising	Presence of bruising is significant and will require specialist advice and examination as it may be indicative of abuse or rape
Circumcision	Female circumcision is not common in the UK but may be seen in some ethnic groups
Parasites	Pediculosis (lice)
	Pthirus pubis (crab louse)
Palpation	
Only required to palpate swellings present, e.g. Bartholin's gland area for enlargement or tenderness	Bartholin's gland infection is usually unilateral (signs are swelling, tenderness, heat or discharge)

Checklist continued

Pelvic examination	
This should not be carried out unless symptomatically indicated	
Using a speculum inspect the	
• Vaginal walls for	
Abnormal nodularity, masses or tenderness	Tumour
	Infection
	Abscess
Assessment of discharge	The colour and consistency of the vaginal secretions may be an indication of infection
	Bleeding may be coming from uterus or vaginal walls
Laxity	Rectocele or cystocele
Vaginismus occurs when there is spasm in the bulbocavernosus muscle, which produces acute pain on examination	
• Cervix	Ectropion
The cervix should be mobile and not tender. Note size, shape and consistency, any tenderness and mobility	Polyps
	Carcinoma
	Cervicitis
Taking a specimen for cervical cytology should only be undertaken after specialist training	
Bi-manual examination	
• Uterus for	Pregnancy
Abnormalities of size	Fibroid
should be 5.5–8 cm long and pear shaped	Tumour
Shape and consistency	Fibroid
	Tumour
Tenderness	Pelvic inflammatory disease
	Endometriosis
Lack of mobility	Fibroid
	Tumour
	Adhesions
	Pregnancy
• Adnexa	
Presence of a mass	Ovarian cysts
	Tumours
	Uncommonly carcinoma of the bowel or diverticulitis may also be palpable
Tenderness	Swollen fallopian tubes in pelvic inflammatory disease
	Ectopic pregnancy: *if ectopic pregnancy is suspected a vaginal examination should not be carried out as it may rupture the tubal pregnancy*

Checklist continued

ANAL AND RECTAL EXAMINATION: REFER TO CHAPTER 5	
PROSTATE EXAMINATION (MALES ONLY) **Rectum**	
Refer to Abdominal examination in Chapter 5 for examination of the rectum	
• Digital examination	
The prostate gland should feel firm, smooth and slightly mobile, and should not be tender.	
Rubbery or boggy consistency	Benign hypertrophy
Stony hard, nodular	Carcinoma
	Prostatic calculi
	Chronic fibrosis
Fluctuant softness	Prostatic abscess

THE EVIDENCE

There is a lack of research relating to examination of the penis and the scrotum in general.

Testicular examination

The evidence base regarding the reliability and examination of the testicles is poor. There is, however, plenty of data available for testicular cancer. Presentation is usually with testicular enlargement or lump and in 97 per cent of these patients a lump is present on examination (Scottish Intercollegiate Guidelines Network 1998).

In 2008, the European Association of Urology produced guidelines on **testicular cancer**. Within this document, they advise screening by self-physical examination in the presence of clinical risk factors because, although the advantages of screening programmes have not been demonstrated via surveys, it has been shown that the stage and prognosis of testicular cancer is directly related to early diagnosis (Albers *et al.* 2009). Testicular cancer is very susceptible to modern treatments and survival for early diagnosis is 95–100 per cent (Austoker 1994).

Daniels and Layer (2003) suggest that there may be a correlation between testicular tumours and **gynaecomastia:** in a small retrospective study, four out of the 127 patients who had gynaecomastia were also found to have a testicular tumour.

Female examination

Pelvic examination is routinely carried out for many reasons to identify or negate pathological problems. However, the literature suggests that it is unwise to base treatment decisions on **bi-manual examination** results alone (Brown and Herbert 2003) and positive findings should be backed up with further assessment. An extensive review of the literature regarding pelvic examination revealed no evidence to support the pelvic examination of asymptomatic women for screening purposes; it has a low sensitivity and specificity for the detection of ovarian malignancy (Stewart and Thistlethwiate 2006). Even in ideal circumstances where accuracy of the pelvic examination was assessed in 140 women under general anaesthetic, the uterine assessment had a specificity of 80 per cent and a sensitivity of 64 per cent, but assessment of adnexal masses was even lower, with a sensitivity of 51 per cent and a positive predictive value of only 43.8 per cent (Padilla *et al.* 2005). Patient characteristics such as obesity, uterine size and abdominal scars make an accurate examination more difficult. The experience of the clinician also has an influence on the examination: in Padilla *et al.*'s study (2005) the overall accuracy of the examination was 70.2 per cent for gynaecologists, 64.0 per cent for residents and 57.3 per cent for medical students.

Another small study of 186 patients by Close *et al.* (2001) concluded that the interobserver reliability of bi-manual examination by emergency doctors was poor. They recommend that although it should not be abandoned clinicians must appreciate its limitations.

The literature is in agreement that carrying out a vaginal examination when **ectopic pregnancy** is suspected is ill advised and a study of 382 patients (Mol *et al.* 1999) with suspected ectopic pregnancy gave good evidence that there was no benefit of carrying out a vaginal examination to confirm an ectopic pregnancy.

Rectovaginal examination is not widely used and in some clinical assessment books it is not even mentioned. Although it is suggested that it is used to detect post-uterine nodularity, a study by Dragisic *et al.* (2003) found that even under ideal conditions (of 140 patients under general anaesthetic) it was poor in the detection of endometriosis. It is not recommended as a technique for general use.

Prostate examination

The evidence of the value of prostate examination is again quite limited, but there is a consensus that **digital rectal examination** is of value both in symptomatic males and also for screening, but must not be used exclusively for diagnosis (Gosselaar *et al.* 2008; Issa *et al.* 2006; Pedersen *et al.* 1990; Smith and Catalona 1995; Varenhorst *et al.* 1992).

 REFLECTION ON PRACTICE

TEAMWORK

An 84-year-old woman (Mrs P) presented to her local pharmacy requesting antibiotics for the treatment of cystitis. The lady was well known to the pharmacist. She lived in the village, and collected her monthly prescription for hypertension regularly. She had been widowed for many years but lived independently and managed well.

She had sought advice from the pharmacist on many issues over the years but was informed by her friend that he could now prescribe her antibiotics. (The pharmacist had become an independent prescriber.)

While taking the history he noted that she had had many similar episodes of cystitis and was regularly given antibiotics for this problem.

He did not have any record of these prescriptions because she usually picked them up from the chemist in town approximately 3 miles away (situated next to the surgery).

She could not recall exactly how often the problem occurred or what medication she had been given; in fact her total recall was very vague. As the pharmacist could not establish an accurate past medical history or drug history he contacted the surgery to speak with the General Practitioner (GP). Although physical examination was normal, he was concerned as her symptoms were significant and urinalysis showed a trace of blood and protein.

During discussion with the GP it transpired that Mrs P had problems with a persistent

continued ➢

REFLECTION ON PRACTICE *continued*

infection which was not clearing despite many courses of different antibiotics and had already been referred to an urologist. They agreed that another mid-stream specimen of urine (MSU) should be sent to the laboratory and that a copy of the result would be sent to the pharmacist; a course of antibiotics was commenced in accordance with the last sensitivity result.

When the result of the MSU was available to the pharmacist, he called Mrs P into the pharmacy and asked her to bring in all the medications that she had at home in order to establish her concordance with previous courses. Mrs P came down to the pharmacy that afternoon with a carrier bag full of medicines. The pharmacist was surprised to see how many medications she had accumulated. When he looked through the bag with her permission he found all the courses of antibiotics that had been prescribed by the GP were still intact in the boxes.

Further questioning revealed that she only took medications that the pharmacist had given her. The others had been collected by her friend from the chemist in town, but she didn't like to offend her.

Mrs P had not taken any of the antibiotics prescribed to her and subsequently her infection was persisting. The intuition of the pharmacist regarding Mrs P's symptoms and poor history alerted him to a more significant problem than cystitis. He discussed this issue with her at length and she said that she was taking the current course that he prescribed. They made arrangements to do another MSU when the course had finished. The pharmacist contacted the GP to alert him of the problem and they agreed that the pharmacist should be alerted if she had any further prescriptions so that he could check concordance.

This story highlights the importance of a good history and teamwork to ensure safe and effective management.

CASE STUDY

42-year-old male

Presenting complaint: Pain and swelling in his scrotum.

History of presenting complaint: Pain started about a week ago, then he noticed a swelling in the left side of his scrotum 2 days ago. Never had any previous problems.

Past medical history: Asthmatic, otherwise nil of note.

Family history: Nil relevant.

Drug history: Asthma inhalers only.

Allergies: Nil.

Social history: Lives with wife and three children and works as builder/bricklayer.

Ex-smoker (smoked for few years as teenager only).

Enjoys alcohol socially only usually at weekends with friends or out with wife (within recommended limits).

Enjoys swimming and goes twice weekly to local pool.

Systems review: Normally fit and well, but feeling tired and achy for the past few days.

Appetite is reduced.
Sleeping more than normal.
No urinary or abdominal symptoms.

Preliminary examination

Looks fit and healthy.
Temperature 36.6°C, pulse 70 beats per minute, respirations 18 breaths per minute, blood pressure 120/60.

Test yourself

1 What are the differential diagnoses for a scrotal swelling?
2 How can you distinguish the difference on examination?
3 On examination you find a scrotal enlargement with a non-tender, cystic swelling anterior to and below his right testicle. The testis is easily palpable, and the swelling will transilluminate easily. What is your most likely diagnosis?

Answers can be found at the back of the book (p. 123).

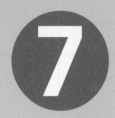

7 THE UPPER LIMB

Zoë Rawles

Shoulder pain can severely compromise a person's activities of daily living and unfortunately it seems that chronic and recurrent problems are common (Winters *et al.* 1999). The examination of the shoulder may be reassuring to the patient and may provide the practitioner with some idea of the problem and how it impacts on the patient's life, and it is therefore useful to become familiar with it. It may also determine the advice given to the patient including recommended activity and the need for physiotherapy referral or joint injection.

There are well over a hundred different tests that can be performed during a shoulder examination. The following procedure list encompasses the main observations and range of movements necessary for a basic examination of the shoulder and upper limb.

Where there is a history of trauma, the joints above and below the affected joint should be examined.

Perform a preliminary examination first (Chapter 1). Of particular importance are the general appearance, vital signs (for the detection of systemic disease), pulse and examination of the hands. Always examine the normal limb first for comparison with the abnormal limb.

CHECKLIST	
PROCEDURE	**RATIONALE/POSSIBLE PATHOLOGY**
SHOULDER EXAMINATION	
With all system examinations a good history is essential and the assessment of the upper limb is no exception. The evidence highlights the importance of the history over physical examination in making a diagnosis	There are many possible causes of shoulder/upper limb pain that are not necessarily musculoskeletal in origin, e.g. referred pain from abdominal and thoracic sites. Consider angina, ectopic pregnancy, cholecystitis, etc Diabetes mellitus, inflammatory arthritis, breast surgery, or chest surgery may predispose to adhesive capsulitis
Assess the neck function observing for full range of pain-free movement: extension, flexion, rotation, side flexion (Chapter 8)	Referred pain from neck pathology
INSPECT Watch the patient remove clothing and assess for any restricted range of movement (ROM). Both shoulders should be fully exposed Inspect both shoulders from front, side and behind	

Checklist continued

Look for	
• Asymmetry or deformity, e.g. winging of scapula	Weakness of the serratus anterior resulting from injury to the nerve
• Wasting, e.g. of supraspinatus or infraspinatus muscles	Rotator cuff tear in the elderly person
	Neurological deficit
• Swelling: assess the type	
Fluctuant	Build up of synovial fluid due to inflammation or trauma
Firm/hard	Cystic/bony/nodular
Boggy	Haemarthrosis (*bleeding in the joint*) due to trauma or clotting disorder
	Pyarthrosis (*pus*), e.g. septic arthritis
• Scars	Surgery
• Bruising	Injury
• Dislocation	
• Rash	Sepsis or specific skin problem with associated joint pathology, e.g. psoriatic arthropathy (*an association between psoriasis and joint disease*)
• Erythema	Inflammation and/or infection
PALPATE	
Use a systematic approach	Location of the pain may aid diagnosis
Anteriorly	
Over sternoclavicular joint, clavicle, acromioclavicular (AC) joint, humeral head, coracoid process	AC pain often arises from joint itself
Laterally	
Over the deltoid muscle	Deltoid pain may be caused by tendonitis, rotator cuff pathology
Posteriorly	
Over spine of the scapula, supraspinatus muscle, infraspinatus muscle, trapezius muscle	
Note	
• Hot areas (using back of hand)	Infection
	Inflammation
• Tenderness	Arthritis
• Swelling	Gout
	Effusion
• Wasting of muscles (*using finger tips*)	Loss of function
• Crepitus in the joint (*this can be done when checking passive movement by placing a hand over the joint. Crepitus will be felt when two roughened surfaces come into contact*)	Osteoarthritis

Checklist continued

CHECK MOVEMENT (FIG. 7.1)	
Estimate degree of limitation compared with normal side	To be able to identify if the movement on the affected side is actually abnormal for that particular patient
Quantify movements in degrees	
Stand in front of the patient face to face and ask them to copy the movements you make	It is easier to demonstrate these movements than to describe them, although observation of abduction can be done from behind to check for abnormal movement of the scapula, where pain limits true glenohumeral function
Active movements	
Normal degree of movement is shown in brackets	Movements of the shoulder are dependent on five functional areas: glenohumeral joint, acromioclavicular joint, subacromial joint, sternoclavicular joint and scapulothoracic region
Ask the patient to put the arm in the neutral (adduction) position: flexed	
Check	
• Rotation (internal and external) in neutral adduction position	Assessing the range of movement may help to determine the location of the pathology. It will also determine the extent of disability and effect on activities of daily living
• Flexion (180°) and extension (45–60°)	
• Abduction (90° if scapula is held in place by the examiner or 'anchored', increasing to 180° if scapulothoracic movement is allowed)	Anchoring the scapula facilitates a test of true glenohumeral function
• Adduction (45°)	
• Rotation (internal 70–90° and external 90°) in abduction	
Cross-arm test (*forward elevation to 90° with active adduction. Positive if gentle pressure on the joint in this position causes pain*)	Acromioclavicular joint pathology, e.g. arthritis

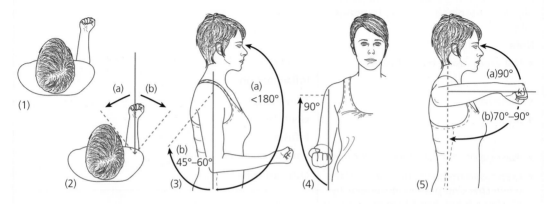

Fig. 7.1. Shoulder – normal range of movement. (1) Adduction in a neutral position; (2) rotation in adduction: (a) internal rotation and (b) external rotation; (3) (a) flexion; (b) extension; (4) abduction (angle is increased to 180° with scapulothoracic movement); (5) (a) external rotation in abduction (e.g. brushing hair); (b) internal rotation in abduction (e.g. doing up a bra).

Checklist continued

Passive movements	
Check the same range of passive movement and compare	
Assess whether	
• Passive movement is less painful	Reduced active movement that improves on passive movement generally indicates a muscular or tendon problem
• Greater range of passive movement in affected limb	Soft tissue injury
• Active *and* passive movement painful and restricted	Joint instability
	Ligament rupture
	Fracture
	Previous injury
	Adhesive capsulitis
	Bony injury
	Dislocation
Other tests	
Check for a 'painful arc': *position arm straight down at side and check active and passive elevation*	
Look for pain in early abduction 60–120°	Rotator cuff lesion due to compression of a damaged or inflamed suprasinatus tendon against the acromial arch, i.e. impingement
	Passive movement here will be less painful because impingement is reduced
Look for pain in a high arc 90–180°	Acromioclavicular pathology, e.g. arthritis
Check the 'drop arm test': *raise the patient's arm to 90°. Ask the patient to hold the arm in that position and then to slowly lower the arm. Observe for sudden dropping of the arm. Check to see if arm gives way when gentle pressure applied (positive test)*	Large rotator cuff tear
Depending on the practitioner's expertise other tests for **impingement** may be performed, e.g.	A test for **impingement** may be useful when pain is exacerbated by activities that involve the arm moving overhead or above the shoulder
• Neer's test	Refer to The Evidence section for a discussion on when and if these tests should be included
• Hawkins–Kennedy test	
• Empty can/full can	
• Copeland impingement test	
• Dawbarn's test	
• Coracoid impingement test	

Checklist continued

ELBOW EXAMINATION	
INSPECT BOTH ELBOWS FROM FRONT/SIDE/BEHIND **Look for**	

• Asymmetry/deformities
  Varus (*inward angulation*)
  Valgus (*outward angulation*)
	Supracondylar fracture
	Non-union of lateral condylar fracture

• Muscle wasting	Loss of function
• Scars/bruising	
• Injury	Portal for infection
• Swelling	Effusion, olecranon bursitis Arthritis
• Inflammation	Gout
• Rash/psoriasis/eczema	Psoriatic arthropathy
• Subcutaneous nodules	Gouty tophi Rheumatoid arthritis
PALPATE Ask about pain before starting **Palpate posteriorly and feel for**	
• Temperature: heat	Inflammation and /or infection

• Swelling
  Soft and fluctuant
  Boggy
  Hard
	
	Fluid: olecranon bursitis
	Synovial thickening as in rheumatoid arthritis
	Bony injury

• Tenderness
  Localized over medial epicondyle
  Localized over lateral epicondyle
	
	'Golfers elbow'
	'Tennis elbow'

CHECK MOVEMENT **Check elbow function** Estimate degree of limitation compared with normal side. Quantify movements in degrees	To rule out elbow pathology as a cause of restricted range of movement in the lower arm
Active movements With upper arm held against the body, check	
• Flexion (normal 150°) and extension (normal 0°)	Tests the joint between the humerus and ulna
• Pronation: *palms facing down* (normal 70°)	
• Supination: *palms up as if holding a bowl of 'soup' for 'soupination'!* (normal 90°)	Tests the radio-ulna joints

Checklist continued

Passive movements	
Check same range of passive movements as for active and compare. Assess whether	
• Passive movement is less painful than active	Soft tissue injury more likely
• Greater range of passive movement in affected limb	Joint instability
	Ligament rupture
	Fracture
	Previous injury
• Active and passive movement painful and restricted	Fracture/bony injury

WRIST AND HAND EXAMINATION	
INSPECT (DORSAL AND PALMAR)	
Assess for	
• Contour and symmetry	
Muscle wasting in hypothenar or thenar eminence	Median or ulnar nerve palsy
Isolated wasting of thenar eminence	Carpal tunnel syndrome
Generalized wasting of small muscles	Rheumatoid arthritis
	Old age
• Rash/skin disorder, e.g. eczema, psoriasis	Psoriatic plaques may indicate a form of psoriatic arthropathy that can mimic rheumatoid arthritis
• Erythema	Gout
	Infection
• Purpuric rash	Vasculitic conditions, e.g. rheumatoid arthritis
• Swelling: distribution	Effusion
• Deformity e.g. swan necking, ulnar deviation (*usually associated with anterior subluxation of the fingers*)	Rheumatoid arthritis
• Dupuytren's contracture	Genetic
	More common in diabetes, alcoholism, epilepsy
• Trigger finger (*finger becomes locked in flexion. It may be due to inflammation and swelling of a tendon or tendon sheath*)	Repetitive movement/strain injury
• Heberden's nodes (*osteophytes at the base of the distal phalanx*)	Osteoarthritis
• Bouchard's nodes (*osteophytes in the proximal interphalangeal joints*)	Osteoarthritis

Checklist continued

PALPATE SYSTEMATICALLY, CHECKING FOR	
• Temperature: heat	Inflammation
	Infection
• Swelling	Fracture
	Ganglion
	Carpal tunnel syndrome
	Pregnancy
	Hypothyroidism
	Lymphoedema
	Numerous other causes. Assess the characteristics of the swelling and remember the history
• Tenderness:	
In 'anatomic snuff box'	Likely scaphoid fracture
	Refer for an X-ray
Around radial styloid	De Quervain's tenosynovitis
70 **Carpal compression test**	
If the history suggests symptoms of carpal tunnel syndrome (i.e. median neuropathy) then perform a carpal compression test by applying pressure with the thumb over the carpal tunnel for 30 seconds to reproduce symptoms	A positive carpal compression test indicates median neuropathy
70 **CHECK MOVEMENT**	
Active and passive movements	To assess the site and severity of the problem
Wrist	To assess the range of movement and possible impact on activities of daily living
• Extension	May indicate a diagnosis
• Flexion	
• Radial and ulnar deviation	
Hand	
• Thumb: basal joint: palmar and radial abduction/adduction	Weak thumb abduction is present in carpal tunnel syndrome
• Thumb: interphalangeal: hyperextension/flexion	
• Thumb: metacarpophalangeal hyperextension/flexion	Hyperextension may be congenital or due to injury
• Finger distal interphalangeal (DIP) joints: extension/flexion	
• Finger proximal interphalangeal (PIP) joints: extension/flexion	
• Finger metacarpophalangeal (MCP) joints: hyperextension/flexion	Hyperextension may be due to dislocation

THE EVIDENCE

Shoulder examination

It is difficult to evaluate the evidence for the diagnostic value of the various components of the shoulder examination. Even where tests can be proven to predict a specific diagnosis (which is not often), what cannot be easily evaluated is how far a diagnosis will actually affect the management. Recent research indicates that over 50 per cent of the tests used in the physical examination of the shoulder did not meet statistical criteria for acceptable reliability (Nomden *et al.* 2009).

Mitchell *et al.* (2005) in a clinical review describe a lack of consensus on diagnostic criteria and methods of assessment that complicates treatment choices. They suggest that the overcomplicated approach to diagnosis is unlikely to alter the early conservative management of shoulder pain.

History

Shoulder pain is a good example of where the history is likely to be more important than the examination. A full history should go some way to excluding the possibility of referred shoulder pain. Referred pain is usually referred distally, felt deeply and does not cross the midline (gp-training.net 2006). Careful questioning should determine how long the patient has had the symptoms, possible aggravating factors and how the symptoms are affecting their life. If the patient is older than 65 years, has pain at night when lying on the affected side and has a history of trauma, then a rotator cuff tear is quite likely (Litaker *et al.* 2000). Occupations involving lifting, repetitive awkward movements and vibrations may be important in provoking or exacerbating impingement. It is thought that inflammation of the tendons caused by contact against the coracoacromial arch can in time create a rotator cuff tear. This seems to be somewhat dependent on age, with less than 1 per cent of shoulder injuries being due to tears in the under 30 year olds compared with 35 per cent in patients older than 45 years with shoulder pain (Stevenson and Trojian 2002).

Rotator Cuff lesions

A review of the evidence states that in order to suggest a diagnosis of rotator cuff tear the most important individual clinical findings are the positive dropped arm test and age equal or over 60 years (McGee 2001). Clinical findings that may argue against this diagnosis are age under or equal to 39 years, absence of painful arc and negative impingement signs.

Impingement

Researching methods for demonstrating the '**painful arc**' revealed numerous different descriptions and techniques but very little evidence to promote one method over another. A study of 125 patients with painful shoulder implied that although various shoulder tests including 'the painful arc' may be helpful with clinical evaluation of the patient, they do not necessarily help with making a diagnosis (Calis *et al.* 2000). A small study of 30 patients similarly concluded that most physical examination tests for impingement may be reasonably good at predicting impingement but that imaging techniques should be recommended where necessary to better define shoulder lesions (Silva *et al.* 2008). A meta-analysis of individual tests concluded that the diagnostic accuracy of the Neer test and the Hawkins–Kennedy test for impingement is limited and described a 'lack of clarity' regarding the various tests in terms of how useful they are to provide differential diagnoses in shoulder pathology (Hegedus *et al.* 2008). It is recommended that practitioners only perform these tests when they are confident that they can achieve a meaningful result and that this may affect their management of the patient.

Hand and wrist

Examination of the elbow and the hand or wrist is not as complicated as for the shoulder and a decision on management may be more straightforward, with surgery an earlier possible option depending on the diagnosis.

Range of movement

Details for examining movement are included in the procedure list, but one study suggests that physical examination of the wrist and hand contributes only a minimal amount of reliable information. Detailed questionnaires may constitute more effective tools for diagnosing wrist and hand complaints (Salerno *et al.* 2000).

Carpal compression test

Evidence for the various tests is often conflicting, with some studies suggesting the tests are useful and others not. One study indicates that Phalen's and Tinel's signs can both be used to check for carpal tunnel syndrome but the carpal compression test has a higher sensitivity and specificity and is therefore likely to be more useful (Moses 2008). It is simple and fast and has been shown to be a very reliable provocative test (González del Pino *et al.* 1997). A systematic review of 12 publications where clinical tests were evaluated with nerve conduction tests as gold standard, concluded that Phalen's and Tinel's signs are not helpful in predicting carpal tunnel syndrome (D'Arcy and McGee 2000). Because of the lack of reliable evidence determining the usefulness of Phalen's and Tinel's tests compared with the carpal compression test, they have not been included in this procedure list.

 REFLECTION ON PRACTICE

WHEN ELBOW PAIN IS NOT WHAT IT SEEMS
Bill Smith was a 60 year old who presented with intermittent pain over the medial epicondyle. It was definitely related to exercise. It had started to come on when he went jogging and he thought it may be to do with the way he held his arm. It also came on when he carried heavy dustbins to the bottom of the drive and sometimes when mowing the lawn. Recently it had been particularly bad when walking upstairs or up a hill. Sometimes the pain seemed to spread into the upper arm and made him stop what he was doing. He occasionally had an associated aching sensation in the left side of his chest. It always subsided after a few minutes rest. He had always been a keen golfer and one of his friends had told him it was 'golfer's elbow' but it did not always seem to come on during his game so he was a little confused and wanted a definite diagnosis.

A full history revealed a past medical history of rheumatic fever but nothing else of significance. On examination there was no tenderness, inflammation or swelling over the epicondyle and Bill had a full range of movement without any problem. Auscultation of the heart seemed normal and there was no palpable apex beat.

A standard electrocardiogram (ECG) and exercise ECG were both normal and a subsequent angiogram showed only mild atherosclerosis in keeping with Bill's age. He was advised by the specialist to take aspirin and a statin as a precautionary measure but was assured that the pain was most likely to be gastric or musculoskeletal in origin. Bill hated going to the surgery but some time later he presented again to the practitioner with increasing pain on exertion which was much worse if the wind was cold. He could not relate it to eating and was reluctant to agree with the idea that it was gastric or musculoskeletal. The pain still started in the elbow and upper arm and the chest pain came on afterwards. He had also had some episodes of dizziness on exertion. This time the practitioner referred him back to secondary care and he was given an echocardiogram. There was evidence of aortic stenosis and it seemed likely that Bill's pain was angina occurring as a result of this.

continued ➤

REFLECTION ON PRACTICE *continued*

He went on to have a valve replacement and his symptoms have since improved.

This story is based on a personal experience and demonstrates the need to consider all possible causes of pain and to be persistent. The practitioner had been concerned about referring Bill back to secondary care having already been advised that this problem was not likely to be cardiac. In the event she was very glad she had tried again. In this instance Bill's echocardiogram may have been delayed because his initial investigations were inconclusive, and presumably the specialist was unable to detect symptoms on auscultation that warranted further tests.

CASE STUDY

55-year-old female

Presenting complaint: Sudden onset of pain and stiffness in the left shoulder 3 days ago.

The pain is disturbing her sleep and she is having problems brushing her hair and dressing. She is off work and is worried as her employers are not sympathetic to employees who have time off sick.

History of presenting complaint: Previously well – no symptoms.

Medical history: Diabetic (Type 2).

Drug history: Metformin, gliclazide, ibuprofen.

Family history: Mum had Type 2 diabetes and died at 74 years. Dad had hypertension and angina and died from a myocardial infarction at 70 years. One brother – hypertension.

Social history: Works as a part-time check-out operator. Happily married. Two grown up children. Drinks alcohol occasionally. Diet is high fat/low fibre. Smoker 20 per day.

Systems review: Nil of note.

Preliminary examination

Appears to be in pain with her shoulder.
Blood pressure: 160/94.
Body mass index: 32.
Nil else of note.

Test yourself

1 When you examine this patient's shoulder you note that passive movements are a little easier than active movement, although all range of movement is limited. There is a negative drop arm test. What might this indicate?

2 Which other test may be helpful here?

3 How will you manage this patient initially?

4 What other factors besides the shoulder pain need to be considered in this case?

Answers can be found at the back of the book (p. 123).

8 THE BACK

Zoë Rawles

Examining the back is fairly straightforward, but there is no particular sign or combination of signs that can be gleaned from the examination that will confirm any particular diagnosis or prognosis following treatment (Bogduk and McGuirk 2002).

The following checklist encompasses the main observations and range of movements necessary for a basic examination of the back.

When there are neurological symptoms a neurological assessment should be performed (Chapter 10).

Patients who have 'red flags' identified from the history require immediate attention and further investigation. (**Red flags** are listed in Table 8.1 in the discussion of evidence.)

 Observe the patient as they walk into the consulting room, the way they walk and how much pain they appear to be in as this may conflict with the history.

Perform a thorough preliminary examination first (Chapter 1).

CHECKLIST	
PROCEDURE	**RATIONALE/POSSIBLE PATHOLOGY**
CERVICAL SPINE (Patient sitting)	
Note that following major trauma the neck should be immobilized and a lateral radiograph obtained	
OBSERVE	
• How the patient moves and holds their neck	Decreased range of movement is common with spasm or pain from any cause
• Anteriorly: for torticollis (*misalignment or twisting*)	May occur where there is acute wryneck, fracture, dislocation, tumour, infection, scar tissue, spondylosis, inflammatory processes, infection. May be idiopathic
• Laterally for normal cervical lordosis (*inward curvature*)	Kyphosis (*abnormal outward curvature*) in the cervical spine is uncommon but may occur in osteoporosis and ankylosing spondylitis (*chronic inflammatory arthritis of the spine and the sacro-ilium that eventually leads to fusion of the spine*)
• From behind, noting any scars, muscle bulk or muscle wasting	Surgery Trauma

Checklist continued

	Poor posture leading to overuse of craniocervical flexor muscles
	Muscle spasm
	Neurological pathology
PALPATE **Each spinous process** **Note any**	
• Prominence/kyphosis	Osteoporosis and ankylosing spondylitis
• Tenderness over a vertebra	Collapsed vertebra, infection or tumour
	Supraspinous damage
• **Tenderness over the cervical spine – midline**	Cervical spine fracture
• Paraspinal tenderness with radiation into trapezius	Cervical spondylosis (*degenerative osteoarthritis in the cervical spine*)
MOVE (ACTIVE MOVEMENTS) • Flexion (chin on chest: normal is 45°) • Extension (look up: normal is 45°) • Lateral flexion (ear on shoulder: normal is 45°) • Rotation (look over shoulder: normal is 70°)	Checking for range of movements in all areas of the spine may determine degree of disability and may serve to distinguish mechanical from non-mechanical pain but may not help confirm a diagnosis
THORACIC SPINE (Patient standing)	
OBSERVE **Laterally and behind for**	
• Exaggerated kyphosis, malalignment of the vertebrae	Osteoporosis
	Ankylosing spondylitis
	Degenerative disc disease
• Scoliosis (*abnormal curvature in the lateral plane*)	Idiopathic
	Postural
	Congenital
	Muscle spasm
	Legs of unequal length
	Neurological disease
	Tumour affecting the vertebrae
	Infection of the vertebral discs
• Scars	Previous surgery
	Injury
PALPATE • Each individual vertebra for tenderness	Collapsed vertebra
	Infection
	Tumour
• Around the spine for muscle spasm	As a cause of, or as the result of pain

75

76

Checklist continued

MOVE (ACTIVE)	
• Flexion	Range of movement as for cervical spine
• Extension	
• Lateral flexion	
• Rotation (*anchor pelvis by putting your hands on either side, ask patient to twist at waist to each side. Alternatively have the patient seated to perform this manoeuvre*)	To stabilize the hips
LUMBAR SPINE (Patient standing)	
OBSERVE **Laterally and from behind for**	
• Loss of normal concave curvature or lordosis	Loss of lordosis may indicate disc disease
• Exaggerated lordosis	Pregnancy
	Obesity
	Fixed flexion deformity of the hips
	Spondylolisthesis (*anterior or posterior displacement of a vertebra, commonly associated with spondylosis*)
• Scoliosis	Possible pathologies listed under rationale for scoliosis in the thoracic spine
PALPATE	
• Each individual vertebra for tenderness	Collapsed vertebra
	Infection
	Tumour
• Paraspinal muscles for muscle spasm	Inflammation
	As a cause or as the result of pain
• Sacro-iliac joints. Perform lateral compression of the pelvis to detect any pain in the sacroiliac joints	Sacro-iliitis as in ankylosing spondylitis, Reiter's syndrome (*reactive arthritis occurring in response to an infection elsewhere in the body*), psoriatic arthritis
MOVE (ACTIVE MOVEMENTS): **As for thoracic spine**	As for cervical/thoracic spine
Note that flexion, extension and lateral flexion of the thoracic and lumbar spine can be difficult to separate	The length of the spine should increase with lumbar flexion
If necessary perform Schober's test to check specifically for lumbar flexion	
Look for reduced lumbar flexion	Ankylosing spondylitis
Schober's test	
• *With patient standing mark the midpoint between the posterior superior iliac spines (located at L5)*	
• *Make a mark 10 cm up from the first point*	
• *Ask the patient to touch their toes*	

76

Checklist continued

• *Re-measure the distance between the two points: this should have increased by >5 cm*	
TESTING FOR NERVE ROOT IRRITATION With the patient lying supine, perform **passive straight leg raises** (SLRs). *If this provokes pain radiating from the back into the buttock and thigh along the sciatic nerve distribution, the test is positive* During SLR pain below the knee at less than 70° is made worse by dorsiflexion of the ankle and is relieved by ankle plantar flexion, suggests tension of the L5 or S1 nerve root related to disc herniation Crossover pain, where pain is aggravated in the affected limb when the unaffected limb is raised, is also a strong indication of nerve root compression	Assesses sciatic nerve compression but many elderly patients will not be able to flex the hip past 70°

76

THE EVIDENCE

Croft (2000) in a *British Medical Journal* editorial discussed the findings of various studies and concluded that in most cases no clear cause for the back pain can be identified. Many tests lack reliability and validity so that clinical signs elicited during examination should be interpreted cautiously. Given this information the practitioner could be forgiven for asking why they need to do a full examination, but there are good reasons. It is reassuring for the patient and illustrates that the practitioner is interested. It also enables the practitioner to check for red flags (Table 8.1) and thereby rule out serious spinal pathology. It can also be useful in terms of monitoring disability in chronic pain. McGuirk *et al.* (2001) compared the safety, efficacy and cost-effectiveness of evidence-based medical care and usual care for acute low back pain. They suggest that while examination of the back does not take long to do, it can serve to identify the exact site of the pain and may eliminate the need for further expensive and unnecessary investigations.

Red flags

All current literature and research support the mandatory checking for 'red flags' when taking a history from and assessing the patient with back pain (Table 8.1).

Where there are 'red flags', the examination of the back should be more thorough and include a neurological assessment and examination of the chest and/or abdomen as appropriate in order to assess for serious pathology: for example, infection, malignancy, neurological compromise or aortic aneurysm.

Tenderness over the cervical spine

It is not within the remit of this book to explore examination of the trauma patient in any depth. However, patients who have been involved in a road traffic accident or other trauma often present some

Table 8.1 Red flags (adapted from information provided by gp-training.net and the EMIS Mentor Authoring Team 2007)

Major trauma, e.g. road traffic accident or fall from a height
Age under 20 or over 55 years
Non-mechanical pain
Thoracic pain
Cancer, steroids, HIV (human immunodeficiency virus) or other significant past history
Unwell, weight loss
Widespread neurology, e.g. bilateral leg signs
Structural deformity
Persistent night pain
Saddle anaesthesia/sphincter disturbance: always record if present, it may indicate possible cauda
  equina syndrome and require emergency admission
Diabetes
Penetrating wounds
Post menopause

time after the event in a non-emergency appointment and the practitioner must be prepared to act accordingly. Heffernan *et al.* (2005), in a single-centre prospective observational study of 406 patients, concluded that spinal tenderness warrants imaging. A study by Gonzalez *et al.* (1999) involving 2176 blunt trauma patients suggests that clinical examination in the awake and alert blunt trauma patient is reliable in determining significant cervical spine injury, although other studies disagree (Duane *et al.* 2007). The absence of midline tenderness does not rule out significant spinal injury (D'Costa *et al.* 2005). Where there is any doubt the practitioner should ensure immediate immobilisation of the patient and request an X-ray of the cervical spine.

Assessing range of movement

A cross-sectional population based study of 4000 people concluded that there was only a weak correlation between the assessment of severity of back pain according to the findings on clinical examination compared with subjectively reported pain and disability (Michel *et al.* 1997).

Littlewood and May (2007) in a systematic review of four relevant studies demonstrated little evidence to support the use of current methods to assess spinal function and degree of impairment. The authors suggest the need for more scientific research to assess the validity of checking for the range of movement.

Until there is more comprehensive research to indicate that assessing the range of movement in the spine is of no value, it should be included in the examination if only to determine the extent of disability and monitor progress.

Passive straight leg raising test

This is included in the procedure list as it is widely used to help diagnose nerve root pain, although a systematic review of published papers between 1989 and 2000 (Rebain *et al.* 2002) describes little consensus on interpretation of results and suggests that more research is needed into the clinical usefulness of passive straight leg raising. A further review by Devillé *et al.* (2000) involving a search of studies conducted between 1992 and 1997 cautiously concludes that straight leg raising tests (specifically the Test of Lasègue) may have a low diagnostic accuracy, although the authors acknowledge that there may be some limitations to the review.

REFLECTION ON PRACTICE

CONSIDERING THE PATIENT HOLISTICALLY

Betty Jones had suffered with intermittent back pain for years having sustained an injury while lifting a patient when she worked as a nurse. It had recently flared up again and this time was not improving as quickly as previously. The practitioner (Bob) had prescribed analgesia and referred her for some physiotherapy. However, Betty kept coming back, the pain was no better and she was beginning to feel quite depressed with it. The analgesia did not help that much, but it did make her constipated. Bob had taken a thorough clinical history and felt confident about dealing with this as there were no 'red flags' indicating the need for referral. He tried many different analgesics without much success. She had been referred for acupuncture and to the pain clinic but the waiting list was long and she was unlikely to get an appointment for some months. One day when exploring Betty's low mood to assess her for potential depression, Betty broke down in tears and explained that she was a carer for her husband who was severely disabled with rheumatoid arthritis. She felt she could no longer cope since having problems with her back and she had no family close by to help.

She had failed to mention this before and her husband was registered with another practice and so he was not known to Bob. She had been reluctant to mention it because her husband was adamant that he did not want to go into a home or have anyone else caring for him and she felt she was letting him down.

After discussing the help that was available with Betty, Bob was able to refer her husband to the Community Nursing Team for assessment. Following this a hoist was supplied and a member of the team visited regularly to build a relationship with Mr Jones until he felt comfortable with them assisting his wife. He also agreed to go into a home for respite care so that his wife was able to have a short break.

Betty's back continued to cause discomfort for some time but despite this she was now able to cope more easily and was happy to have some long overdue help.

It is vital that as practitioners we carefully consider all possible factors in the patient's life and environment that may be causing distress and prolong the healing process. No amount of medication or other treatment will cure a problem where there are underlying, compounding factors.

CASE STUDY

46-year-old female

Presenting complaint: Sharp burning pain in the lower back and right buttock radiating down the side of the thigh and below the knee. Some associated numbness and tingling in the right buttock and thigh. Made worse with sneezing or laughing.

History of presenting complaint: Symptoms for 3 days: started with pain just in the lower back and buttock. Came on a few hours after moving some heavy furniture. Previously well. History of mild intermittent back pain over many years, usually eased with non-steroidal anti-inflammatory medication.

Medical history: One pregnancy to full term 10 years ago. Nil else of note.

Drug history: Paracetamol every 4 hours for the last 3 days.

No herbal or illicit drugs. No allergies.

Family history: Both parents alive and well. One brother 40 years old: well.

Social history: Lives with partner and child. Rented accommodation. Works as a teacher.

No stress or financial concerns. No recent travel. Sleeps well normally but not for the past two nights due to the discomfort. Smokes 10 a day. 10 units alcohol spread throughout the week.

Normal varied diet. Swims occasionally. Enjoys gardening.

Systems review: Nil abnormal.

Test yourself

1 What is the likely diagnosis?
2 Which tests would help to confirm the diagnosis?
3 What other checks should be done during the examination with this patient?
4 Suggest the likely non-pharmacological management and prognosis.

Answers can be found at the back of the book (p. 124).

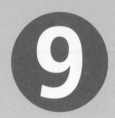

THE LOWER LIMB

Beth Griffiths

Start with observation as the patient enters the room; the way they are walking, weight bearing and how much pain they appear to be in. Observation when the patient is not aware is vital for this examination. Sometimes the level of pain observed differs from the history.

Always compare with the other side and examine the unaffected limb first. This gives a more reasonable comparison for the patient's normal range of movements especially in older people. If more than one joint is involved then all of the major joints should be assessed to detect systemic disease. If there is a history of trauma, the joints above and below the affected area should be tested.

Motor and sensory testing must also be carried out if neurological involvement is suspected (refer to Chapter 10). Disease of the neurological system can also affect muscle response, tone and power. If there is any evidence of a vascular problem then all the major arteries should be palpated and auscultated as described in the Cardiovascular Examination (Chapter 2).

Perform a preliminary examination first. Of particular importance are gait, general appearance, vital signs (detection of systemic disease), pulses and hands.

CHECKLIST

PROCEDURE	RATIONALE/POSSIBLE PATHOLOGY
KNEE **Inspect for**	
• Alignment (*the angle between the tibia and the femur should be less than 15°: commonly called the Q angle*)	Knock knees (genu valgum) or bow legs (genu varum) may be present, can be congenital or acquired, e.g. osteoarthritis causes bowing
• Deformity	Flexion contractures commonly found in intrinsic knee disease
• Scars	Previous surgery or injury
• Atrophy of quadriceps, hamstring and calf muscles	Indicates wasting of the local muscles from lack of use or neurological disease
• Loss of normal hollows around patella	An early sign of swelling or fluid in the joint
• Any swellings in or around the knee	Bursitis over the patella or anserine bursitis
	Baker's cyst in the popliteal area.
	Effusions of the knee joint may be seen if large

Checklist continued

Palpate	The location of the tenderness can be an indication of the problem
• Along joint line	Can be suggestive of **meniscal tears**
• Medial and/or lateral side of knee, extending above and below the joint	Collateral ligament injury or can be present in morbidly obese patients
• Medial femoral condyle	Osteonecrosis (*loss of blood supply to the bone causing necrosis*)
• Medial tibial plateau	Bursitis, stress fracture of the plateau or osteonecrosis
• Over the patella	Pre-patellar bursitis, especially if warm and inflamed
• Popliteal space	Baker's cyst
Tests for effusion	
• The Bulge sign	Useful for detecting small effusions only
• Ballottement test (*useful for intermediate effusions*) *When the patella is separated from the femur by fluid, the sharp thrust makes it collide against the femur. If no fluid is present the patella will be sitting against the femur and no click will be heard*	Effusions can be due to synovial fluid, blood or pus

They may be caused by injury, systemic disease, or infection |
Range of movement (ROM) (Fig. 9.1) *While carrying out passive movements note any crepitus in the joints*	Can be a sign of degenerative joint disease if painful, but also present in a normal joint if not painful
Specific tests for ligament injuries	
• Medial and lateral collateral ligaments	
Pain	In either ligament could indicate ligament injury
Instability of the joint	Could indicate rupture of the collaterals, meniscus or **cruciate ligaments** and warrants further investigation
• Lachman test	If the tibia moves excessively forward it indicates subluxation and instability of the anterior cruciate ligament
• Anterior drawer test (*a positive test results in an unrestrained forward motion*)	Detects a possible tear of the anterior cruciate ligament
• Posterior drawer test (*a positive test results in an unrestrained backward motion*)	Detects a possible tear of the posterior cruciate ligament

Fig. 9.1. Range of movement of the knee.

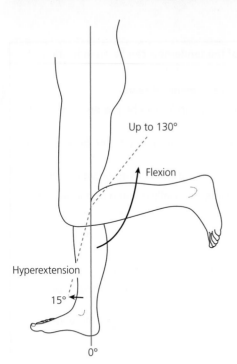

Checklist continued

HIPS
Inspection
With patient standing, and walking, check for
 	
• Alignment
Trendelenburg gait occurs when the pelvis on the opposite side drops and the body leans away from the affected side while weight bearing on the affected hip
 	
Supine on the bed check for
 	
• Leg length
 	
• Deformities
• Is there rotation of the foot
 	
• Scars
	
	Caused by
	   Muscle weakness
	   L5 compression
	   After poliomyelitis
	
	Leg shortening is commonly seen in fractured neck of femur
	Congenital or previous injuries
	External rotation is commonly seen in fractured neck of femur
	Previous surgery

Checklist continued

Palpate the	
• Greater trochanter for tenderness	Soreness may indicate bursitis
• Ischial tuberosity	Ischiogluteal bursitis
Range of movement	
See Fig. 9.2 for all ranges of movements	
Ask patient to flex hip and carry out other movements passively	
• Flexion	Pelvic tilting could indicate fixed **flexion** deformity
• Extension	
• Abduction and adduction	Restricted abduction is common in hip disease
• Internal and external rotation	Can be an indicator of hip disease such as osteoarthritis
ANKLE AND FOOT	
Inspection	
Ask patient to walk on toes or stand on one leg and raise heel off the floor	This assesses the integrity of the motor system and helps to exclude neurological involvement
• Foot and ankle alignment from in front and behind	Gives clues about problems with gait originating from other areas, e.g. back or hips
• Check shoes for signs of abnormal wear	

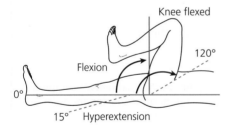

Fig. 9.2. Range of movement of the hip.

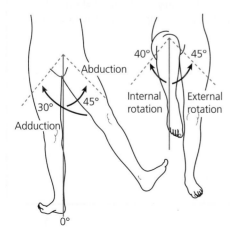

Checklist continued

• Note arch height	Pes planus (flat feet) *occur when the longitudinal arch flattens so that the sole of the foot approaches or touches the floor*
	Pes cavus occurs when the arch is abnormally high
• Deformity or callosities	Hammer
	Claw toes
	Hallux valgus (bunion)
• Inflammation	May indicate gout or cellulitis
• Swelling	Around an area of injury could indicate fracture or haematoma
• Verrucas	May be painful and causing altered gait
Palpate	
• Ankle joint for	
Bogginess, swelling or tenderness	Arthritis
	Injury
	Stress fracture
	Infection
• Achilles tendon for	Rheumatoid nodules
Nodules and tenderness	Achilles tendnitis
	Achilles bursitis
	Tendon xanthoma
	Retrocalcaneal bursitis
• Metatarsophalangeal (MTP) joints for	
Bony tenderness	Injury
	Early sign of rheumatoid arthritis
If joint is inflamed	Gout
	Infection
Morton's neuroma (*press together the heads of the second and third metatarsals and then the third and fourth*)	Reproduction of the pain on this manoeuvre suggests Morton's neuroma (*entrapment of the common digital nerve between the metatarsal heads*)
Test for tarsal tunnel syndrome. *If symptoms suggestive of nerve entrapment, percuss over the nerve below and posterior to the medial malleolus*	Pain, numbness and burning on the medial side of the foot, ankle or calf indicates tarsal tunnel syndrome
Soft tissue (tenderness in the plantar soft tissue)	Plantar fasciitis
Range of movement (Fig. 9.3)	
An arthritic foot is usually painful in all directions, but in ligament injuries the pain is reproduced when the ligament is stretched	

Fig. 9.3. Range of movement of the foot.

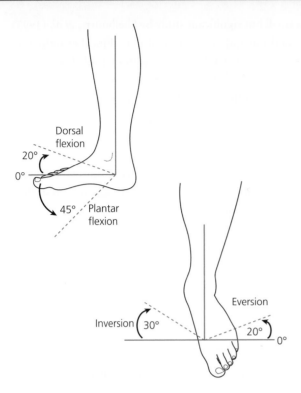

THE EVIDENCE

Range of movement

McGee (2001) found in his review of the evidence that range of movement testing in any joint is one of the most sensitive indicators of joint disease.

Tests for ligament injury in the knee

Solomon *et al.* (2001) conducted a literature review from 1966 to 2000 and found no adequate evidence for the diagnostic accuracy of manoeuvres to test the integrity of the collateral ligaments. They assert that a composite examination (good history and several clinical tests) for specific meniscal or ligament injuries of the knee performs much better than specific manoeuvres. They also suggest that synthesis of a group of examination manoeuvres is required for adequate diagnosis.

Lachman test

Testing for **cruciate ligament** injury has been more thoroughly researched. A review of the evidence by Davis (2002) found the Lachman test to be the most accurate but also the most difficult to perform correctly.

In another review of the evidence, Jackson *et al.* (2003) suggest that the Lachman test has a mean sensitivity of 84 per cent and specificity of 100 per cent (when performed by orthopaedic specialists).

The **posterior drawer test** also had a sensitivity of 91 per cent and specificity of 98 per cent.

The **anterior drawer test** had a sensitivity of more than 82 per cent and specificity of more than 94 per cent. The anterior drawer test is not as accurate as the Lachman test but it is easier to perform.

Testing for meniscal tears is less accurate. In a small but significant study by Shelbourne *et al.* (1995) sensitivity and specificity were found to be low and the authors concluded that clinical examination alone cannot determine the location, shape or length of the tear. In patients with multiple knee lesions the accuracy of testing is less reliable and has been found to be as low as 30 per cent.

Mangione (2008) adds that these tests have predominantly been replaced by the magnetic resonance imaging (MRI) scan for a definitive diagnosis.

Tests for hip movements

The evidence relating to specific tests for hip examination is poor, except for a small study by Peeler and Anderson (2007) that assessed examination of **hip flexion**. Although it is a commonly used test, they question the reliability of the Thomas test, and suggest that further research is needed.

Although specific tests are not well researched a small study by Cibere *et al.* (2008) indicates that a comprehensive hip examination (including the above-mentioned manoeuvres) can be performed with adequate reliability for assessment of osteoarthritis.

 REFLECTION ON PRACTICE

EXPECT THE UNEXPECTED

A 48-year-old gentleman presented in the surgery requesting the drug naproxen for gout. He was referred to the Nurse Practitioner (NP) for assessment. It was on Friday afternoon and the previous week a patient in the surgery who was being treated for gout in a foot joint had been diagnosed with a deep vein thrombosis (DVT), so the NP was not complacent about the patient's diagnosis. The patient had previously been treated for gout in his foot 2 years before. This time he felt it was in his right knee. He was systemically well. He described the pain as throbbing and the knee to be warm. On examination the knee was not inflamed or warm and the only abnormality found was a small effusion. He was unable to hyperextend the knee.

The NP carried out a thorough examination and explained to the patient that it was unlikely to be gout in view of the absence of inflammation, and arranged follow-up to investigate the cause of the effusion. The naproxen was issued, as a non-steroidal anti-inflammatory drug was appropriate for the pain and there were no contraindications. A blood sample was taken to check the uric acid level.

Two days later the results were reported to the NP and the uric acid level was reported as 0.56 mmol/L (for men >0.4 mmol/L is hyperuricaemia), which is indicative of gout. She contacted the patient to check on his condition and inform him of the uric acid level and found that he was feeling much better and the knee was almost pain free. Although she had seen gout many times and felt comfortable with its diagnosis, this case demonstrates the importance of listening to the patient as well as using experience and knowledge when treating patients.

CASE STUDY

36-year-old female

Presenting complaint: Pain in the sole of her left foot.

History of presenting complaint: The pain started a few weeks ago but was getting worse over the past week. She is using her father's walking stick to help her walk. There is no history of injury but she is a keen rambler and walks on rough ground regularly. The pain is predominantly in the sole of the foot and is worse when she gets out of bed and starts walking, and again at the end of the day after work. There is no inflammation on the foot.

Past medical history: Nil relevant.

Family history: Nil relevant.

Medication: Nil, no allergies.

Social history: Married, has four children, works as a hairdresser. Non-smoker; occasional alcohol. Body mass index is 32.

Systems review: Nil relevant.

Test yourself

1 List the common causes of foot pain.
2 Thinking about the differential diagnoses for foot pain, which aspects of the history help to correlate to each of these differential diagnoses?
3 What would you look for on examination and why?

Answers can be found at the back of the book (p. 124).

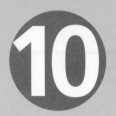

10 THE PERIPHERAL NERVOUS SYSTEM

Trudy Alexander

Ensure that the patient understands what you are going to do and how they are expected to respond in order to eliminate errors through misunderstanding.

Proceed at a pace that is comfortable for the patient as a full nervous system examination can be tiring.

Always test and compare both sides of the body.

Carry out a preliminary examination first. Particular attention should be paid to vital signs, skin, wasting and the tongue (B12 deficiency).

CHECKLIST

PROCEDURE	RATIONALE/POSSIBLE PATHOLOGY
Analyse the patterns that emerge from the history and the examination	To determine the site of the lesion
	To determine the likely pathology
	Many disease processes can affect any part of the nervous system. These include tumours, infections, demyelination such as in multiple sclerosis (Fig. 10.1), injury, bone disorders, congenital disorders, hereditary disease, vascular disorders, degenerative disorders, toxicity and metabolic disorders
OBSERVE GAIT Watch the person walk normally, on heels, on toes and 'tightrope' walking **Brain**	
• Festinating gait which is slow and shuffling	Parkinson's disease
• Hemiplegic gait in which the patient swings the leg around to step forward	Cerebrovascular accident
• Diplegic gait in which the patient's legs are circumducted	Bilateral lesions close to the ventricles
• Choreiform gait with irregular, jerky, involuntary movements	Some basal ganglia disorders such as Huntington's chorea
• Ataxic gait with wide-stepping, irregular, lurching steps and truncal instability	Cerebellar disease (and severe loss of proprioception)
• Scissors gait	Cerebral palsy
• Spastic gait with stiffness and dragging of the foot	Brain abscess, tumour, trauma and cerebrovascular accident

93

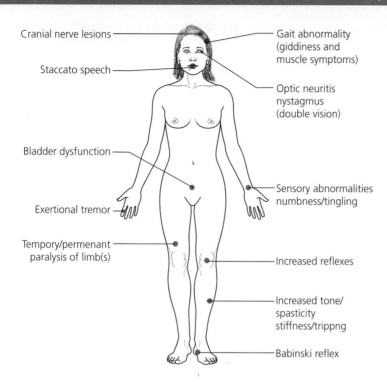

Cranial nerve lesions

Staccato speech

Bladder dysfunction

Exertional tremor

Tempory/permenant paralysis of limb(s)

Gait abnormality (giddiness and muscle symptoms)

Optic neuritis nystagmus (double vision)

Sensory abnormalities numbness/tingling

Increased reflexes

Increased tone/ spasticity stiffness/trippng

Babinski reflex

Fig. 10.1. Signs associated with multiple sclerosis.

Checklist continued

Spinal cord • Scissors gait	Cervical spondylosis, trauma and tumours. Caused by nerve root compression
• Neuropathic high-stepping gait	Lumbar disc protrusion
Peripheral nerves • Neuropathic high-stepping gait	Peripheral neuropathy
• Any gait abnormality	Multiple sclerosis may affect any part of the nervous system and could therefore result in an assortment of gait abnormalities (Fig. 10.1)
	Musculoskeletal disorders, vestibular disorders, age, foot problems and visual problems
PERFORM ROMBERG'S TEST A test for joint position sense. *The patient is steady with the eyes open but unsteady with them closed because the eyes compensate for loss of position sense*	Posterior spinal cord lesions such as cervical spondylosis and tumours (Fig. 10.2, the posterior column in the spinal cord which relays joint position sense) Peripheral neuropathy
If the patient is unsteady with the eyes open other diagnoses should be considered	Vestibular disorders Cerebellar disorders

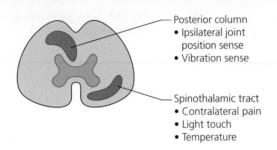

Posterior column
• Ipsilateral joint position sense
• Vibration sense

Spinothalamic tract
• Contralateral pain
• Light touch
• Temperature

Fig. 10.2. Sensory tracts in the spinal cord, from the right-hand side of the body.

Checklist continued

TEST FOR THE ABILITY TO MAINTAIN POSTURE The application and prompt release of downward pressure to outstretched upper and lower limbs. The limb may oscillate if abnormal	Cerebellar disorders
CARRY OUT TESTS FOR COORDINATION Observe for inability to carry out movements involving rapid repetition of the upper and lower limbs	Cerebellum Impaired position sense Muscle weakness Visual disturbance
INSPECT THE LIMBS FOR • Temperature, colour, skin texture • Rash • Scars • Wasting of muscles • Symmetry • Fasciculation • Involuntary movement • Bone or joint deformity	The following examples are a selection of the many possible abnormal findings Shiny hairless skin in peripheral neuropathy Purpuric rash in meningitis Operations or injuries resulting in nerve damage Lower motor neurone lesion such as nerve root dysfunction Differences that highlight problems such as wasting Lower motor neurone disorders such as motor neurone disease Upper motor neurone disorder such as Huntington's chorea Charcot joint in peripheral neuropathy

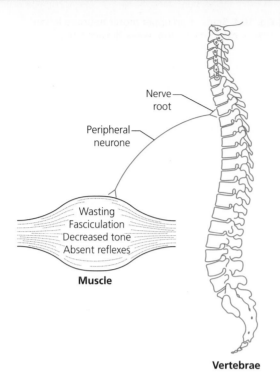

Fig. 10.3. Signs of a lower motor neurone lesion.

Nerve root

Peripheral neurone

Wasting
Fasciculation
Decreased tone
Absent reflexes

Muscle

Vertebrae

Checklist continued

TEST FOR MUSCLE TONE IN ALL LIMBS Normally there will be slight resistance to passive movement	
In complete loss of tone the limb will be flaccid	
• Reduced tone	Lower motor neurone lesions (Fig. 10.3). Disease affecting the cerebellum Myopathies The acute phase following a cerebrovascular accident (spinal shock)
• Spasticity (sudden increased tone)	Usually an upper motor neurone lesion (Fig. 10.4) The chronic phase of a cerebrovascular accident *In a cerebrovascular accident of the frontal lobes and in dementia increased tone resembles resistance on the part of the patient*
• Lead pipe rigidity (generally increased tone) and cogwheel rigidity (tone intermittently increased at regular intervals)	Usually pathology affecting the extrapyramidal tracts such as: Parkinson's disease Drugs, e.g. phenothiazines

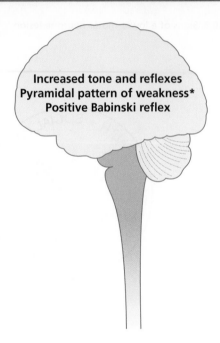

**Increased tone and reflexes
Pyramidal pattern of weakness*
Positive Babinski reflex**

Fig. 10.4. Signs of an upper motor neurone lesion.
*Weak extensors in arm; weak flexors in leg.

Checklist continued

TEST POWER IN THE LIMBS	
Knowledge of the muscles, nerves and nerve roots that are involved in carrying out movements helps to determine the location of the lesion. The pattern of weakness combined with findings from the rest of the neurological examination will help to determine whether the cause is an upper motor neurone lesion, a lower motor neurone lesion, muscle disease, disease involving the neuromuscular junction or functional weakness	Fig. 10.4 (pattern of weakness in an upper motor neurone lesion)
• Weakness in all four limbs	A lesion in the cervical spinal cord or bilateral pyramidal tracts, e.g. trauma, transverse myelitis
• Weakness in arm and leg on the opposite side of the lesion	A lesion in one cerebral hemisphere, e.g. cerebrovascular accident
• Weakness in a single limb	A lesion affecting one cerebral hemisphere, the brainstem, spinal cord, nerve root or a single nerve, e.g. hand weakness in an ulnar nerve lesion
• Variable weakness	Neuromuscular junction disease, e.g. myasthenia gravis

Fig. 10.5. Reflexes.

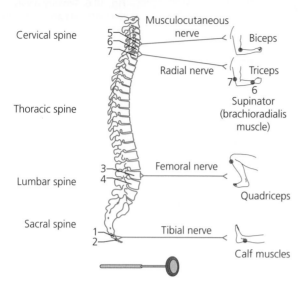

Musculocutaneous nerve
Cervical spine
5
6
7
Biceps
Radial nerve
Triceps
7
6
Supinator
(brachioradialis
muscle)
Thoracic spine
Femoral nerve
Lumbar spine
3
4
Quadriceps
Sacral spine
1
2
Tibial nerve
Calf muscles

Checklist continued

TEST THE REFLEXES (FIGS 10.3–10.5) Use reinforcement techniques such as the Jendrassik manoeuvre when it is difficult to elicit a reflex Observe for abnormal reflexes, and other abnormal responses such as the involvement of other muscles, slow relaxing muscles or repeated contraction of the muscle	
• Decreased or absent reflexes	Lower motor neurone lesions. These are lesions that involve the peripheral nerves or the nerve roots
Biceps jerk	Musculocutaneous nerve, nerve root C5 (C6)
Triceps jerk	Radial nerve, nerve root C7
Supinator jerk	Radial nerve, nerve root C6 (C5)
Knee jerk	Femoral nerve, nerve root L3–L4
Ankle jerk	Tibial nerve, nerve root S1–S2
• Increased/brisk reflexes	Upper motor neurone lesion. These are lesions that involve the brain or the spinal cord
	In the acute phase of an upper motor neurone lesion, such as a cerebrovascular accident or spinal cord compression, reflexes may however be absent. This is due to spinal shock
• Babinski response	Upper motor neurone lesions, e.g. spinal cord compression, cerebrovascular accident
	Sensory abnormalities, weakness and the withdrawal response could affect the outcome
• Any abnormal reflex	Musculoskeletal abnormalities or incomplete relaxation

94

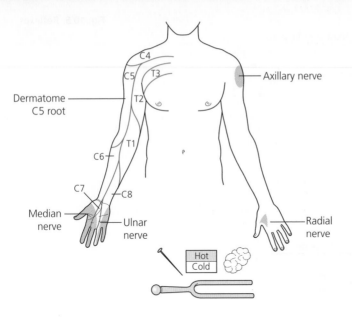

Fig. 10.6. Sensory areas: dermatomes and individual nerves.

Checklist *continued*

CARRY OUT TESTS FOR SIMPLE SENSATION Light touch Pain Vibration sense Temperature Joint position sense Sacral sensation if the history or examination suggest possible cauda equina syndrome	*Sensory loss might be found in a particular dermatome or an area supplied by an individual nerve (Fig. 10.6). Two different pathways in the spinal cord transmit sensation. The posterior column transmits joint position and vibration sense whereas the spinothalmic tract transmits pain, light touch and temperature. Lesions in either pathway can therefore result in the loss of different sensations. Different patterns may therefore emerge depending upon the site of any lesion (Fig 10.2, p 88)*
Brain • Contralateral sensory loss	Lesions in either cerebral hemisphere or the thalamus, e.g. cerebrovascular accident
• Unilateral sensory loss in the face and part of the opposite side of the body	Brainstem injury
Spinal cord • Sensory loss below the lesion	A complete spinal cord lesion, e.g. injury
• Sensory loss involving both arms and hands	Lesions of the central cord, e.g. syringomyelia (cavities surrounded by proliferation of connective tissue)
• The Brown–Séquard syndrome (pain and temperature sensation are lost on one side, whilst the sense of touch is lost on the opposite side)	Lesions involving half of the cord
Radiculopathy • Sensory loss in the corresponding dermatome	Nerve root irritation, e.g. disc protrusion

Checklist continued

Individual nerves	
• Sensory loss in the feet and hands	Polyneuropathy, e.g. diabetes mellitus
• Sensory loss in the distribution of the median nerve	Carpal tunnel syndrome
CARRY OUT TESTS FOR CORTICAL SENSATION: These include two point discrimination, tactile recognition of objects, graphaesthesia, localization of sensation, simultaneous bilateral tactile stimulation and perception of weights The cortex interprets these sensations and the tests are therefore only useful if the simple sensations are intact • Altered sensation in the opposite distal limbs	 Lesions of the posterior parietal lobe

THE EVIDENCE

The physical signs of neurological disease are well researched, unlike the reliability of the actual techniques used to detect these signs. The studies that are available suggest that the neurological examination is still crucial. However, attributes of the patient such as inattention and attributes of the examiner such as inexperience both affect the reliability of the examination (Hansen *et al.* 1994a,b). This is particularly true for the neurological examination, which can be lengthy and requires considerable concentration and cooperation between the examiner and the patient. The patient must therefore be as relaxed and comfortable as possible and must understand how they are expected to respond throughout. Accuracy is improved if the examination is performed when neither the examiner nor the patient is tired.

Practice and a good underpinning knowledge of neurology are fundamental.

Analysis of the patterns that emerge from the history and examination

Anderson *et al.* (2005) in a study involving 46 patients and 16 control subjects found that the interpretation of findings is not always accurate, particularly in early cerebral disease. When all the components of the neurological examination were considered in unison, focal brain disease was detected in 61 per cent of patients. Studies of the reliability of tests for muscle strength (Jepsen *et al.* 2004), sensation (Jepsen *et al.* 2006a) and also the accuracy of diagnosis (Jepsen *et al.* 2006b) suggested fair to moderate agreement between two examiners for 41 patients. Larger, more rigorous studies would be needed to test the validity of these findings. In a slightly larger study involving 99 patients diagnosed with spinocerebellar ataxia a standard neurological examination scoring system was used to test the reliability of the examination and also agreement between examiners (Kieling *et al.* 2008). The scoring system was found to be a reliable measure of disease severity in this type of patient. Various scoring systems have also been developed to detect diabetic polyneuropathy. Costa *et al.* (2006) tested a protocol involving pinprick, tuning fork, monofilament, ankle jerk, cold spatula and walking on heels in 80 patients and 45 control subjects. It was found that isolated signs and symptoms could not identify those with polyneuropathy but those with higher degrees of impairment could be identified using this scoring system. Although these studies are small, there is a trend that suggests improved reliability when the individual components of the neurological examination are considered collectively.

The ankle jerk

Various positions are used to test the reflexes but very few studies have examined whether this affects sensitivity. Oluwole *et al.* (2001) used three examiners to test the ankle jerk in 21 healthy volunteers. The effect of hip abduction, hip adduction and the kneeling position was compared. Sensitivity was found to be best with the patient kneeling, and abduction was found to be better than adduction. Insufficient studies tackling the variations in neurological examination techniques have been carried out to draw any conclusions or to make recommendations regarding which are the most reliable.

 REFLECTION ON PRACTICE

THE PRACTITIONER'S EMOTIONAL RESPONSE TO PATIENTS

It had been a hectic morning and when the practitioner saw that the next person on her patient list was Mr Grimshaw her heart sank. Mr Grimshaw was an angry man and seeing him always made her feel anxious. He suffered from asthma/chronic obstructive pulmonary disease (COPD), having previously been a heavy smoker. He also suffered from chronic low back pain. The practitioner knew that he was probably coming to see her again because of an infective exacerbation of his COPD, which usually needed to be treated with oral steroids as well as antibiotics. This was in fact the case. She examined his chest as quickly as possible and prescribed the appropriate treatment. Mr Grimshaw also requested a repeat prescription for analgesia as his back pain had become much worse due to coughing. The practitioner had noticed that he had difficulty in moving around because of the pain and hastily issued the prescription.

The next day the practitioner was upset to learn that Mr Grimshaw had been admitted as an emergency suffering from cauda equina syndrome. Had she checked for new symptoms, she would have been prompted to carry out a neurological examination, and found evidence of cord compression. Mr Grimshaw had many risk factors for osteoporosis, which increased the possibility of vertebral collapse.

This story demonstrates the importance of checking for changes before issuing repeat prescriptions and of checking for 'red flags'. The story also demonstrates the effect of the practitioner's emotional response on the consultation. Practitioners should be aware of these emotions in order to prevent negative responses that could be detrimental to patient care.

 CASE STUDY

34-year-old male

Presenting complaint: Neck stiffness and pain. No neurological symptoms.

History of presenting complaint: There had been wet weather warnings on the weather forecast on the day that the patient went to court. He desperately wanted joint custody of his children and the inner turmoil meant that he had slept poorly the night before. Smartly

continued ➢

dressed in a suit and tie he was ready an hour early and decided to have some coffee to keep him alert. Fatefully he spilt coffee on his shirt and had to change it at the last minute. Driving a little too fast through the darkness and into the lashing rain he skidded on a bend in a country lane. The car became stuck in the mud at the side of the road. He escaped seemingly unhurt and a passer-by was kind enough to take him to his destination. It was the next evening before the patient started to feel the aches and pains. His neck was very stiff and sore so he made an appointment with the private physiotherapist who had treated his knee in the past.

Past medical history: Meniscal tear 3 years ago.

Medication: Ibuprofen as required.

Family history: Mother osteoarthritis.

Social: Recently divorced sports teacher. Alcohol 20 units a week. Rugby player.

System review: Nil.

The initial examination reveals that there is no midline cervical tenderness or obvious deformity. The patient is comfortable in a sitting position. Athletic build. A healthy body mass index.

Test yourself

1 When should a physical examination be excluded?
2 If on examination active rotation to the right and left is significantly reduced, how should the examiner proceed?
3 Is this patient at high or low risk of significant injury and why?
4 What is the likely diagnosis?
5 What other health assessment might be made?

Answers can be found at the back of the book (p. 125).

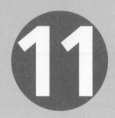

11 THE CRANIAL NERVES

Trudy Alexander

The neurological examination requires more concentration from the patient than any other examination. For this reason, it is vital that the patient understands what is going to happen and how they are expected to respond.

Some examination techniques are highly specific. It should however be borne in mind that the cranial nerve examination is not specific for neurological disorders. For example, abnormalities in strength or movement could be the result of a muscular disorder while abnormalities in visual fields or visual acuity could be caused by disease of the eye itself.

Cranial nerve disorders, in particular, may occur in patients who already have pre-existing disease and this can confound the results of the examination. For example, diabetes is a risk factor for both eye disease and cranial nerve disorders. One should therefore not rule out a cranial nerve disorder simply because a positive finding can be explained by an eye disorder.

Carry out a preliminary examination first. Pay particular attention to vital signs, facial expression and the tongue (twelfth cranial nerve lesion).

CHECKLIST

PROCEDURE	RATIONALE/POSSIBLE PATHOLOGY
It is common for groups of nerves to be affected rather than just one. It is therefore more likely that a lesion will be identified if a thorough examination of all the nerves is carried out Examine each cranial nerve in turn (Fig. 11.1)	Any nerve can be affected by Multiple sclerosis Diabetes mellitus Tumours Sarcoid Vasculitis Syphilis
EXAMINE THE FIRST CRANIAL NERVES (OLFACTORY) A pair of sensory nerves relaying the sense of smell from the nose to the olfactory bulb. The sense of smell is closely linked to taste and therefore taste may also be impaired	

102

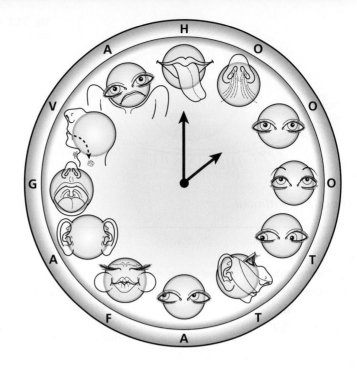

Time	Cranial nerve
12 O'clock	– Hypoglossal
1 O'clock	– Olfactory
2 O'clock	– Optic
3 O'clock	– Occulomotor
4 O'clock	– Trochlear
5 O'clock	– Trigeminal
6 O'clock	– Abducens
7 O'clock	– Facial
8 O'clock	– Auditory
9 O'clock	– Glossopharyngeal
10 O'clock	– Vagus
11 O'clock	– Accessory

Fig. 11.1. The 12 cranial nerves.

Checklist continued

Check smell using the three-item test. Observe for • Anosmia • Parosmia	Trauma Frontal lobe tumour Chronic meningitis Parkinson's disease Refer to Chapter 4 for conditions affecting the nose or sinuses
EXAMINE THE SECOND CRANIAL NERVES (OPTIC) (FIG. 11.2) A pair of sensory nerves relaying the sense of vision from the retina to the visual cortex in the occipital lobes. The nerves from each eye cross over and divide at the optic chiasm before reaching the visual cortex. The site of the lesion will therefore determine which visual fields are lost Assess for defects in • **Visual acuity** using a Snellen chart	 Refractive errors. A pinhole can be used to eliminate this Eye disorders. Refer to Chapter 12 Pre-chiasmal optic nerve lesions such as multiple sclerosis, syphilis or tumours

102

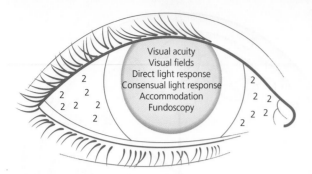

Fig. 11.2. Examination of the second cranial nerves (optic).

Visual acuity
Visual fields
Direct light response
Consensual light response
Accommodation
Fundoscopy

Checklist continued

• **Visual fields** using a confrontation test	
• **Central vision** using a red target	
Defect in one eye	Eye disorder or lesion of the nerve before the optic chiasm, e.g. giant cell arteritis, multiple sclerosis
Defects in both eyes	More likely to be caused by a cranial nerve lesion than disease of the eye
Constricted visual field, arcuate scotoma, altitudinal defect, central scotoma (a scotoma is a blind area)	Disease of the anterior optic nerve, e.g. optic neuritis caused by demyelination, syphilis, collagen vascular disorders
	Retinal lesions
Bitemporal hemianopia. Outer half of visual fields lost in both eyes	Lesions in the optic chiasm including pituitary tumours and internal carotid artery aneurysm
Homonymous hemianopia. Outer half of the visual field lost in one eye and the inner half in the other	Lesions after the optic chiasm such as cerebrovascular accident, abscess, tumour. The majority of lesions that occur after the optic chiasm are lesions of the temporal, parietal and occipital lobes rather than the optic nerve
• Direct light response/consensual light response	
The swinging flashlight test	
The test for accommodation	
Argyll Robertson pupils. Pupils that constrict in response to accommodation but not to light	Wernicke's encephalopathy caused by vitamin B1 deficiency associated with alcohol
	Infections including tertiary syphilis
	Tumours
Adie's pupil. No response to light or accommodation initially. Eventually responds slowly to accommodation and then radiates slowly	Benign and associated with oversensitivity to mydriatic drops
Marcus Gunn pupil/afferent papillary defect. One eye dilates in response to light in the swinging flashlight test	Optic neuritis caused by demyelination, syphilis, collagen vascular disorders
	Large retinal defect
Fixed dilated pupil. No accommodation	Early sign of third cranial nerve lesion. *Constriction and dilatation of the pupil also involves the third cranial nerve (autonomic nervous system)*

Checklist continued

Small pupil with defective dilatation in the dark and ptosis	Horner's syndrome
Difference between pupils	Normal variant
• The retina by carrying out fundoscopy (refer to Chapter 12)	
EXAMINE THE THIRD, FOURTH AND SIXTH CRANIAL NERVES (OCULOMOTOR, TROCHLEAR AND ABDUCENS) Mainly motor nerves relaying impulses from the midbrain to the muscles of the eye and eyelid *If the muscles do not work in synchrony the images fall on different parts of the retina in each eye, which results in diplopia* Inspect and compare both eyes Check cross lateral gaze (eye movements) Observe for	
• Large pupil, ptosis, and difficulty with upward movement resulting in a downwards and outwards deviation	Oculomotor nerve lesion
• Head tilt and difficulty in moving the eye downwards when it is abducted	Trochlear nerve lesion
• Difficulty with outward eye movement	Abducens nerve lesion
• Nystagmus	Oculomotor nerve lesion Cerebellar lesion Vestibular lesion Lesions may be due to ischaemic infarcts, tumours, giant cell arteritis, aneurysms and trauma
• Any defect in movement	Conditions affecting the muscles such as myasthenia gravis or thyroid myopathy Idiopathic
EXAMINE THE FIFTH CRANIAL NERVES (TRIGEMINAL) This pair comprises both sensory and motor components. They originate in the pons varolii and have three branches that supply the face Inspect the face Check muscle power in the jaw Check facial sensation Check for the presence of a corneal reflex	

Checklist continued

This reflex is sometimes absent in normal individuals and is therefore only useful if other abnormalities are found Observe for • Asymmetry, jaw muscle weakness, impaired facial sensation, absent corneal reflex • Numb chin syndrome • Hutchinson's sign. Vesicles on the tip of the nose	 Herpes zoster Bulbar palsy. (Degeneration of the motor cranial nerves) Acoustic neuroma Trigeminal neuralgia Metastatic carcinoma Herpes zoster of the ophthalmic division
EXAMINE THE SEVENTH CRANIAL NERVES (FACIAL) This pair is predominantly motor nerves which originate in the pons varolii. They supply the facial, scalp and neck muscles, lachrymal and salivary glands. The lesser sensory component is involved in taste along with the ninth and tenth cranial nerves Observe facial expression and symmetry Test facial muscles bilaterally Tests for taste can be performed if further testing is thought to be necessary Observe for • Facial paralysis with sparing of the upper face. May occur unilaterally on the opposite side of a lesion • Unilateral facial paralysis. Bell's palsy	 An upper motor neurone disorder such as a cerebrovascular accident A lower motor neurone disorder caused by Polio Otitis media Fractures Herpes zoster Lyme disease (*transmitted by a tick bite*)
EXAMINE THE EIGHTH CRANIAL NERVES (AUDITORY) This pair of sensory nerves is concerned with balance (vestibular branch) and hearing (cochlear branch). *Balance is not affected in slow-growing lesions as the brain adapts* Inspect the external auditory canal and tympanic membrane to check for disorders not related to the cranial nerves	 Refer to Chapter 4 for diseases of the ears, nose and throat

Checklist continued

Test hearing by using the whisper test Observe for • Impaired hearing	Noise Paget's disease Ménière's disease Herpes zoster Acoustic neuroma Cerebrovascular accident of the brainstem Neurofibroma Lead poisoning Drugs such as furosemide, aminoglycosides and aspirin
If any abnormality is detected perform Rinne and Webber tests. Refer to Chapter 4	

EXAMINE THE NINTH AND TENTH CRANIAL NERVES (GLOSSOPHARYNGEAL AND VAGUS)
These nerves originate in the medulla oblongata. The motor component is concerned with swallowing while the sensory component is concerned with taste
Observe for
• Voice/cough abnormalities
  Deviation of the uvula
  Swallowing difficulty
  An abnormal gag reflex and taste disturbance on the posterior third of the tongue. The gag reflex and tests for taste need only be performed if an abnormality is suspected
• A bovine cough
• Swallowing difficulty and a bubbly voice
	
	Bilateral cerebrovascular accident
	Trauma
	Brainstem pathology
	Polio
	Guillain–Barré syndrome. Ascending paralysis usually starting in the lower limbs
	
	Vocal cord palsy
	Tenth nerve lesion

EXAMINE THE ELEVENTH CRANIAL NERVES (ACCESSORY) This pair of nerves originates in the medulla oblongata and the cervical portion of the spinal cord. They supply the trapezius and sternocleidomastoid muscles. They are motor nerves tested by assessing muscle function Inspect the neck and the shoulders Test strength in the shoulder and neck muscles	 Refer to Chapters 7 and 8 (upper limb and back) for musculoskeletal disorders

Checklist continued

Check for	
• Asymmetry	Polio
• Muscle wasting	Syringomyelia
• Weakness	Cerebrovascular accident
	Bulbar palsy
	Trauma
EXAMINE THE TWELFTH CRANIAL NERVES (HYPOGLOSSAL) This pair of motor nerves originates in the medulla oblongata and supplies the muscles of the tongue Check the tongue for • Fasciculation • Wasting • Grooving on one side • Deviation • Weakness	Disease of the cerebral hemispheres, brainstem, or peripheral nerve such as: Metastatic carcinoma Tumours in the neck Trauma Polio Syringomyelia Tuberculosis Thrombosis

THE EVIDENCE

Many studies exist that explain the disease processes affecting the cranial nerves but very few examine the reliability of the examination.

Olfactory nerve

A 224-patient study comparing the **three-item smell test** with a well-validated 40-item test concluded that it had a good negative predictive value and is therefore very useful for ruling out lesions (Jackman and Doty 2005).

Visual acuity

Although the Snellen chart is universally accepted for testing visual acuity, several studies have demonstrated that there are faults in the design and that it can be unreliable (McGraw *et al.* 1995). Various other charts have been designed, but at present their validity has not been demonstrated. The Snellen chart is therefore the one that is currently recommended, but if visual changes involve two lines or fewer the examiner should be cautious when interpreting the findings (McGraw *et al.* 1995). The correct distance and lighting conditions are essential for reliability (Pandit 1994).

Visual fields

Different confrontation tests have been compared with each other and with computerized perimetry (Bass *et al.* 2007; Shahinfar *et al.* 1995; Johnson and Baloh 1991). There is general agreement that confrontation tests are useful in identifying dense visual field defects but not small, shallow defects. Confrontation testing does not have a good negative predictive value as it is relatively insensitive. However, when a visual field defect is identified with confrontation it is usually real. It therefore has a good positive predictive value. Pandit *et al.* (2001) compared perimetry with seven confrontation tests in 138 patients. **Testing central vision with a red target** was the most sensitive examination. The confrontation test is therefore useful but it has many limitations and the results should be interpreted accordingly. Poor examiner technique and lack of understanding on the part of the patient have the potential to affect the reliability of this examination. The examiner should be conversant with the technique being used and the patient must understand what is expected of them.

REFLECTION ON PRACTICE

THE IMPORTANCE OF EVIDENCE-BASED PRACTICE

It was 20 years since Mr Jeffries had been diagnosed with Type 2 diabetes; he always took his medication because he had been told how important this was by the clinical staff at his local surgery, whom he trusted implicitly. As with the rest of this small rural community his family had taken all their concerns to the staff there for the last 35 years. They were always kind and helpful and knew the local families well.

Lately Mr Jeffries had been feeling quite tired and he had developed tingling and pains in his feet which he attributed to standing all day. When his vision became blurred he visited the surgery. He was referred immediately and was diagnosed with proliferative diabetic retinopathy resulting in a vitreous haemorrhage and also peripheral neuropathy. Mr Jeffries was unable to continue his job as a postman and later he lost his home as he could not keep up his mortgage payments.

The healthcare staff in the surgery had not had any diabetes education for many years. The care that they gave was based upon outdated practices and rituals. It was what they had always known and what they felt comfortable with. Educational courses were also difficult to access because of the rural location of the surgery. Mr Jeffries therefore had not had regular screening for his diabetes and his risk factors were not controlled. He was unaware of the fact that his blood pressure, blood sugar and cholesterol were raised and of the significance of this. Consultations were paternalistic and patients were poorly informed about diabetic control. It is possible that Mr Jeffries complications may have been prevented or delayed had the staff at the surgery been more aware of current evidence and he had been more involved in his own care.

This story demonstrates the importance of the need for healthcare professionals to keep themselves updated in accordance with their regulatory obligations. Outdated practices may compromise the wellbeing of patients.

CASE STUDY

60-year-old black African male

Presenting complaint: Weakness in the right side of the face that has apparently resolved.
Occurred 10 days ago and lasted for a day.
A relative observed that the weakness was accompanied by a gait disturbance.

Past medical history: Hypertension.
Myringoplasty following frequent episodes of otitis media.
Intermittent ear infections.

continued ➢

CASE STUDY *continued*

Medication: Amlodipine 10 mg daily

Family history: Father died from heart disease aged 70 years.
  Sister suffers from hypertension.

Social history: Gave up smoking 5 years ago. Smoked 20/day for 35 years.
  Alcohol 21 units a week approximately.
  Divorced with two grown up children and four grandchildren.
  Moved to the UK from Africa with his parents as a child.
  Works as a travel consultant.

Systems review: Slight discomfort in both ears.

Preliminary examination

Blood pressure: 180/100.
Body mass index: 30.

Test yourself

1 List the possible differential diagnoses prior to examination?
2 What examination will you carry out (integrated)?
3 What will you look for to confirm or refute your initial differential diagnoses?

Answers can be found at the back of the book (p. 126).

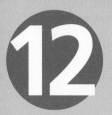

THE EYE

Trudy Alexander

Always consider the more serious although less common causes when taking a history and examining the patient with an eye problem. **Misdiagnoses and delays in treatment** can result in adverse events including **loss of sight**.

Many systemic and autoimmune disorders affect the eye and this should be borne in mind. Consider for example rosacea, sarcoidosis, inflammatory bowel disease and systemic lupus erythematosus. In addition, the probability of serious eye disease is increased in diabetes mellitus and hypertension.

Neurological causes should be considered, as lesions anywhere from the optic nerve to the visual cortex may also cause eye symptoms.

Carry out a preliminary examination first, paying particular attention to blood pressure, temperature and skin rashes.

CHECKLIST

PROCEDURE	RATIONALE/POSSIBLE PATHOLOGY
EXAMINE THE FRONT OF THE EYE, THE ORBIT, THE FACIAL SKIN AND LYMPH NODES (FIG. 12.1) **Observe for**	
• A unilateral red eye	Viral, bacterial and allergic conjunctivitis Spontaneous subconjunctival haemorrhage Acute glaucoma Iritis Episcleritis Scleritis Keratitis Corneal ulcer Foreign body Chemical burn Injury
• Bilateral red eyes	Viral, bacterial and allergic conjunctivitis Keratitis
• Ciliary flush, unilateral	Iritis Keratitis Corneal ulcer Glaucoma

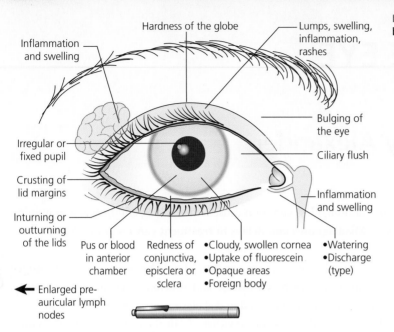

Fig. 12.1. Eye signs that may be found on examination.

Hardness of the globe

Inflammation and swelling

Lumps, swelling, inflammation, rashes

Bulging of the eye

Irregular or fixed pupil

Ciliary flush

Crusting of lid margins

Inflammation and swelling

Inturning or outturning of the lids

Pus or blood in anterior chamber

Redness of conjunctiva, episclera or sclera

• Cloudy, swollen cornea
• Uptake of fluorescein
• Opaque areas
• Foreign body

• Watering
• Discharge (type)

← Enlarged pre-auricular lymph nodes

Checklist continued

• Discharge or pus	Bacterial infection, including Chlamydia trachomatis and gonorrhoea
	Other types of bacterial conjunctivitis
	Keratitis
• Irregular pupil	Iritis
• Fixed semi-dilated pupil	Injury
• Hazy cornea/corneal oedema	Acute glaucoma
• Opaque area on cornea	Acute glaucoma
Stain with fluorescein and examine with a colbalt blue light. Staining allows corneal ulcers to be illuminated	Keratitis
	Contact lens overuse
	Fuchs' endothelial dystrophy
	Eye surgery
	Trauma
	Corneal ulcer
	Dendritic ulcer caused by herpes simplex which is sometimes associated with cold sores
• Epiphoria	Iritis
	Blocked or malpositioned tear ducts
	Abrasion
	Corneal ulcer
	Non-bacterial conjunctivitis
	Ingrowing eyelashes
	Dacryocystitis

Checklist continued

• Hypopyon	Complication of penetrating injury
	Corneal ulcer
	Keratitis
• Hyphaema	Injury
• Object anywhere in the eye	Foreign body
High-velocity foreign bodies such as metal may have penetrated the globe and may not be visible	
• Rash around the eye or on the face	Zoster ophthalmicus associated with herpes zoster
	Corneal ulcer associated with herpes simplex, rosacea, eczema or molluscum contagiosum
• Lumps and other skin lesions	Meibomian cyst
	Hordeolum
	Squamous and basal cell carcinoma
	Melanoma
• Swelling and erythema of the eyelids and surrounding tissue	Orbital cellulitis (pre- or post-septal)
	Allergy
• Erythema and swelling of the inner eye	Dacryocystitis
• Erythema and swelling of the upper outer eye	Dacryoadenititis
• Erythema and crusting of the lid margins	Blepharitis
• Exopthalamus	Hyperthyroidism
	Tumour
	Orbital cellulitis
• Asymmetry of the rim of the orbit and crepitus in the tissues	Blow out fracture following trauma
• Turning out of the eyelashes	Ectropion
• Turning in of the eyelashes	Entropion
Palpate for	
• Enlarged pre-auricular lymph nodes	Viral conjunctivitis
• Hardness of the globe	Acute glaucoma

Checklist continued

102	**TEST VISUAL ACUITY (CHAPTER 11)**	
	• Note any abnormalities or deviation from the patient's norm	Refractive errors
		Corneal disorders such as keratitis
	Refer to Chapter 11 for further information	Glaucoma
		Cataracts
		Iritis
		Retinal detachment
		Vitreous haemorrhage
		Retinopathy
		Maculopathy
		Tumours
		Neurological lesions
		Infections such as cytomegalovirus or toxoplasmosis
		Congenital disorders
103	**TEST VISUAL FIELDS (CHAPTER 11)**	
	Refer to Chapter 11 for further information	
	• Unilateral visual field defects which usually do not cross the horizontal midline	Often due to eye disorders
	• Bilateral visual field defects which usually do not cross over the vertical midline	Often due to neurological lesions
	• Tunnel vision	Advanced glaucoma and retinitis pigmentosa
	TEST DIRECT LIGHT RESPONSE, CONSENSUAL LIGHT RESPONSE AND ACCOMMODATION	
	• Look for abnormal responses	Trauma
		Acute-angle closure glaucoma
		Iritis
		Surgery
		Congenital disorders
		Large retinal lesion
	Refer to Chapter 11	Neurological lesion
	• Poor convergence on accommodation	Thyroid ophthalmopathy
	TEST EYE MOVEMENTS	
	Refer to Chapter 11	
	• Observe for abnormalities such as poor coordination of the eyes or restricted movement	Orbital cellutitis
		Trauma
		Muscular disorders such as myasthenia gravis
		Neurological disorders
	• Observe for nystagmus	Vestibular disorders
		Cerebellar disorders
		Cranial nerve disorders

Checklist continued

FUNDOSCOPY, FIG. 12.2

LOOK FOR THE RED REFLEX • Reduced or absent red reflex *The red reflex is a reflection from the retina and indicates that the pathway from the cornea to the retina is clear. Leukocoria occurs where there is complete absence of the red reflex*	Corneal lesions Cataracts Vitreous haemorrhages Retinoblastoma Retinal detachment
EXAMINE THE DISC OUTLINE, COLOUR, ELEVATION AND VESSELS **Observe for** • Cupping of the disc • Papilloedema • Papillitis • Disc pallor *Optic atrophy*	Glaucoma Tumours Infection Haemorrhage Central retinal vein occlusion Thyroid eye disease Malignant hypertension Optic neuritis Multiple sclerosis Temporal arteritis Tumours Exposure to toxic substances

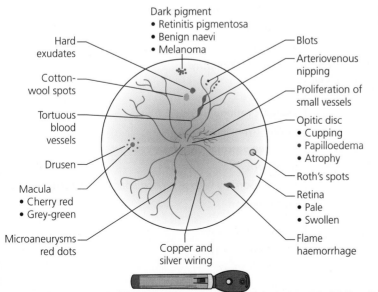

Fig 12.2. Fundoscopy signs.

Checklist continued

EXAMINE THE BLOOD VESSELS IN THE SUPERONASAL ARCADE, THE INFERONASAL ARCADE, THE SUPEROTEMPORAL ARCADE AND THE INFEROTEMPORAL ARCADE **Observe for**	
• Arteriovenous nipping	Chronic moderate and severe hypertension
Occurs when an atherosclerotic-thickened artery crosses over a vein	Left ventricular hypertrophy
• Copper and silver wiring	Hypertension
The artery wall itself is transparent. As the artery becomes thickened the column of blood is smaller and more light is reflected from its surface giving it the appearance initially of copper and then with further thickening of silver wiring	Ageing
• Abnormal branching and formation of new blood vessels.	Diabetic retinopathy Haemoglobinopathies
(In response to retinal ischaemia)	
• Haemorrhages from delicate new blood vessels	Hypertension Diabetes
Potential visual loss if bleeding occurs in the region of the disc or the macula	
EXAMINE THE RETINAL BACKGROUND **Observe for**	
• Cotton-wool spots	Hypertension
Fluffy white areas that are infarcts of nerve fibres	Diabetic retinopathy
	Severe anaemia
	Leukaemia
	Systemic lupus erythematosus
	Infections
• Hard exudates	Hypertension
Off-white or yellow plaques consisting of plasma proteins and lipids that leak from atherosclerotic blood vessels	Diabetic retinopathy
• Dots and blots	Diabetic retinopathy
Red dots are microaneurysms	Severe hypertension
Blots are slightly bigger than dots. They are small haemorrhages in the deeper layers	Collagen vascular diseases
	Infections
	Blood disorders such as severe anaemia and leukaemia
• Flame haemorrhages	Hypertension
These are superficial haemorrhages. When found near the disc they could be associated with papilloedema and raised intracranial pressure, or glaucoma	

Checklist continued

• Retinal detachment *May be visible depending upon its position. Bleeding into the vitreous may obscure the view*	Predisposing conditions include: diabetes, hypertension, myopia
• Vitreous haemorrhage	Diabetic retinopathy Sickle cell anaemia Injury
• Clumps of dark pigment	Retinitis pigmentosa Benign naevi Melanoma
• Roth's spots *Haemorrhages with pale centres*	Leukaemia Diabetes Subacute bacterial endocarditis Pernicious anaemia Human immunodeficiency virus (HIV) retinopathy
EXAMINE THE MACULA **Observe for** • Drusen *Very small round yellow or white patches of extracellular material*	Normal in advancing age
Drusen around the macula	Age-related degenerative maculopathy
Grey-green discolouration, haemorrhages and exudates	Wet-type degenerative maculopathy. *Leads to scarring of the retina*

THE EVIDENCE

Although the majority of the evidence originates from small, non-randomized, uncontrolled studies that may contain bias and cannot be generalized, they contain common themes. The main messages extrapolated from the available evidence were that the accuracy of procedures is improved with appropriate training and that knowing when to refer is critical if adverse outcomes are to be prevented.

Training

Jackson and Glasson (1998) in a study of Australian Primary Care General Practitioners (GPs) found that preventable blindness can be reduced in the community by investing in training and using protocols. Jackson *et al.* (2002) found that after a short workshop, the percentage of GPs able to recognize diabetic retinopathy rose from 24 per cent to 94 per cent.

Fundoscopy

Many studies have focused upon the screening of diabetic patients as they are a large group with significant risk of developing eye complications. Over the years screening methods have become more intricate and extensive, with mass patient recall systems being developed and digital imaging becoming more sophisticated. Clearly mass screening with digital imaging is preferable, but the use of fundoscopy can still be useful. This has been demonstrated in areas where the population has limited access to eye care services (Verma *et al.* 2003) or patients fail to attend their appointments for retinopathy screening (Gill *et al.* 2004).

Misdiagnoses and delays in treatment

Where doubt exists regarding the diagnoses, early referral is essential. Statham *et al.* (2008), in an Australian study involving the audit of 1062 records of patients presenting to the eye emergency services, found that 11 patients had preventable severe adverse outcomes. Ten patients had been diagnosed with conjunctivitis and were treated with chloramphenicol eye drops. Various pathologies, including acute uveitis, keratitis, herpes zoster ophthalmicus, acute glaucoma and retinal detachment, were finally diagnosed and four patients suffered visual loss as a consequence. A correct initial diagnosis was made in only 35.9 per cent of cases referred by GPs, 41.9 per cent of patients referred by emergency department doctors and 48.2 per cent in patients referred by optometrists. Individual cases of missed diagnoses have also been described in the literature. Chang *et al.* (2008) cite the case of a missed intralenticular foreign body, and Gordon-Bennett *et al.* (2006) cite three cases of missed acute-angle glaucoma. Various studies also cite the unnecessary use of chloramphenicol and the resulting delays in care (Sheikh and Hurwitz 2005).

Overall, the evidence suggests that examiners should be adequately trained and clear about their competence before performing eye examinations. Use of the ophthalmoscope requires practice and fundoscopy is sometimes not sensitive enough to locate important pathologies. Routine digital retinal screening for diabetics is the examination of choice if available. The accurate diagnosis of eye disorders requires equipment such as slit lamps, and also adequate time. If the practitioner suspects that the condition is not a benign condition such as conjunctivitis or blepharitis then immediate advice or referral should be sought. Urgent referral should be considered where there is pain, photophobia or blurring of vision (Statham *et al.* 2008).

 REFLECTION ON PRACTICE

RECOGNIZING PERSONAL LIMITATIONS
Peter Gitty enjoyed his new job in the minor injuries unit. He was a qualified Nurse Practitioner and had worked as a Senior Nurse in orthopaedics for several years prior to this. For the first week Peter had been working alongside the Nurse Specialist. Today she was absent because she was unwell and Peter was left to cope with a demanding workload. He had informed his manager that he was alone and that he was inexperienced in this area. Unfortunately, no one was available to cover the Nurse Specialist's absence.

Mr Baker was one of the patients that day. He called in after his shift at the garage where he worked as a mechanic and asked if someone could remove a foreign body from his eye. Peter had seen this procedure carried out and felt that it was something he could tackle. The upper lid was successfully everted and a speck of rust removed.

Mr Baker was however admitted for removal of a penetrating foreign body a few weeks later when his visual acuity deteriorated.

This story demonstrates the importance of recognizing our limitations. Peter did not appreciate the risk associated with the patient's employment because of his inexperience in that particular area. Extended roles and the blurring of boundaries between the roles of

continued ➢

REFLECTION ON PRACTICE *continued*

different healthcare workers have changed the way healthcare is delivered. Within this context it is crucial that the practitioner is aware of his/her own capabilities in terms of education, experience and competency for any work they undertake. The story also highlights the pressures and conflicts that may arise in the workplace. Regulatory bodies stipulate that we are accountable for our actions and omissions. In order to avoid mistakes such as this, various tools can be used such as reflection and clinical supervision. They support the development of self-awareness, assertiveness and the management of difficult situations.

CASE STUDY

18-year-old female

Presenting complaint: The patient had taken a gap year to travel around Australia and was returning to England after having been sky-diving and deep-sea diving in the previous 2 weeks. Her right eye had been sore for a few days but as the aeroplane approached its destination it became quite painful, her vision became blurred and she developed photophobia. Feeling unable to continue her journey home she took a tube train to the hospital where she was quickly triaged and referred to the ophthalmologist.

Past medical history: Myopia. Contact lens wearer. Mild anaemia. Mild acne.

Medication: Diannette.

Family history: Paternal grandmother suffers from type 2 diabetes mellitus. Mother is hypothyroid.

Social history: Non-smoker. Alcohol normally within 14 units weekly but more while in Australia.

Systems review: Nil.

Test yourself

1 What are your differential diagnoses at this stage?
2 What signs might you look for on examination?
3 What examination would be carried out to detect damage to the cornea?
4 What aspects of the history are pertinent and why?

Answers can be found at the back of the book (p. 126).

13 MENTAL HEALTH EXAMINATION

Beth Griffiths

Mental illness can take many forms and dealing with human thoughts, feelings and cognitive functioning is very complex, with a huge variation between individuals. Diagnosing and managing the more serious mental illnesses requires specialist input in most cases, but can be identified and in mild to moderate cases can be treated by a generalist.

There are five main categories of illness: delirium, dementia, mood disorders, psychoses and anxiety disorder, and within this spectrum there are many levels. There are also people who do not have a clinical illness but may have personality traits that resemble some aspects of mental health illness. In these cases the problems are usually chronic and the patient should always be assessed for mental illness by a specialist team before classification.

Organic illness may precipitate mental illness and as such should always be ruled out with an appropriate examination and further investigations when necessary. For example, fever and infection often precipitates delirium in older people. Pathological brain disease such as a tumour, vascular problems and/or trauma can cause personality disturbance. Chronic misuse of alcohol can cause impaired memory and hallucinations. Misuse of recreational drugs such as amphetamines, cocaine and others can produce many signs of mental illness such as hallucinations, delusions and paranoia states. Thyroid and adrenal dysfunction can cause a depressive or manic state. Conversely depression may also be caused by chronic illness and is much more prevalent in patients with a chronic disease.

Assessment of behaviour, thoughts, feelings and cognitive function can be complex and must be related to the person's ability to communicate. For example, if there is a language barrier, or if the patient is illiterate or has learning difficulties, it will affect the outcome of any assessment and allowances must be made within the testing criteria.

There are many different tools that can be used in the mental health examination, but like all assessments the history remains the most important part of the assessment. The mental health assessment should be almost completely incorporated into the context of the consultation with the patient and relative if appropriate. It is very important to consider the patient's narrative before starting more specific questioning in this examination. When specific questioning is required, it should be introduced tactfully and respectfully, with a clear explanation in language the patient can understand. Assessment of the risk of self-harm, suicide or harm to others is a critical part of the examination.

CHECKLIST

MENTAL HEALTH EXAMINATION	RATIONALE/POSSIBLE PATHOLOGY
The mental health status of the patient is generally assessed during the history taking, but there are some specific examination sequences that are required to assess for declining cognitive function, mental illness and depression	
OBSERVE • Level of consciousness If the patient is conscious, their state of alertness and awareness of their environment should be noted	Loss of consciousness is indicative of extensive impairment of the cerebral cortex Changes in attention, memory, orientation and perception can be indicative of acute illness, especially in older people, but also of declining cognitive function or pathological disease
• Posture and motor behaviour	Tense posture, anxiety, fidgeting, crying, pacing, hand wringing are signs of agitation that can be seen in depression Hopelessness, slumped posture and slowed movements are also signs in depression Bizarre behaviour is common in schizophrenia, and mania
• Dress, grooming and hygiene	Deterioration in grooming and hygiene may occur in depression, schizophrenia and organic brain syndromes, but always take into consideration personal norms Excessive fastidiousness can be seen in obsessive–compulsive disorder
• Facial expression and eye contact	Inappropriate expression may be a sign of any of the above Poor eye contact is common in depression
• Manner, affect and relationships	Anger, hostility, suspiciousness or evasiveness can be evident in paranoid states Elation and euphoria can be evident in manic states Flat affect and remoteness are present in schizophrenia Apathy can be present in organic brain disease
• Speech and language	Slowed speech in depression, rapid loud speech in manic states When there are speech and language problems it is important to determine whether it is due to language or aphasia
• Ability to pay attention and participate in the conversation	The inability to engage and participate in conversation may indicate a memory, cognitive or mood disorder and will require further assessment

Checklist continued

MOOD	
To screen for **depression** ask the following questions:	Alteration in mood is very important and can be a normal reactive process. The severity and effect on the person's day-to-day activities must be assessed to determine a deviation from normality. Many patients perceive their low mood or unhappiness to be depression, so objective assessment is important
	Recurring episodes of depression require different strategies for management and depression alternating with mania/euphoria is indicative of bipolar disorder
• Over the past 2 weeks have you felt down, depressed or hopeless? • Over the past 2 weeks have you felt little interest or pleasure in doing things?	If the answer to either one or both of these questions is yes, then further assessment must be carried out
Diagnostic checklist	
• Disturbed sleep • Disturbed appetite	Two or three of the items outlined in this checklist may indicate mild depression
• Guilt or low self-worth • Pessimism or hopelessness • Fatigue or loss of energy • Agitation or slowing of movement	Four or more indicate moderate depression and seven or more with or without psychotic symptoms indicate severe depression
• Diurnal mood variation • Poor concentration • Suicidal thoughts or acts • Loss of self-confidence • Sexual dysfunction	For further information on tools see **Websites for tools**
THOUGHTS AND PERCEPTION	
Does the patient exhibit any delusions, hallucinations, incoherence, bizarre behaviour or paranoia?	Psychotic symptoms indicate gross impairment in reality testing Specialist opinion should be sought when psychosis is suspected
MEMORY, ATTENTION AND COGNITIVE FUNCTION	
• Is the patient orientated to time and place? • Can they remember where they live? • Are they able to read a short sentence? • Can they count back five numerals from 10? • Point out three items and ask them to remember them a few minutes later	If a problem is suspected, testing may be carried out to assess suitability for referral according to local protocol. It is important not to delay referral if the results are only borderline or negative and the history suggests a problem, as early diagnosis is very important

Checklist continued

For more detailed assessment the following tools can be used • **Mini-Mental State Examination (MMSE)** • **6CIT Kingshill Version 2000** • **Abbreviated mental test score (AMTS)** • **Clock drawing test**	The **Mini-Mental State Examination (MMSE)** is considered to be the gold standard for the identification of dementia but it is not useful for screening, or for detecting mild or early dementia. It has been superseded by other tools Refer to The Evidence section for details of these tools
ANXIETY NICE CG22 (2007) gives algorithm guidance for generalized anxiety disorder and panic disorder recognition and treatment	Anxiety disorders are very common and are often intermingled with other mental problems but can exist alone Examples of anxiety disorders are post-traumatic stress disorder, adjustment disorder, panic attacks, agoraphobia and claustrophobia

THE EVIDENCE

Assessment of depression

The **two simple questions** (quoted in the procedure list) about mood and anhedonia are very effective for screening (Arroll *et al.* 2003; MeReC 2001; Whooley *et al.* 1997).

The **diagnostic checklist** is drawn from the World Health Organization (WHO) (2004) guide to depression in primary care. It can be used alone or in conjunction with a tool that scores the severity of the condition.

The literature comparing multiple tools is sparse, this may be due to the nature of the diagnostic problem. There is however consensus that the tools are useful but that diagnostic confirmation must be accompanied by a clinical interview, which then improves the diagnostic accuracy (Williams *et al.* 2002). It is recommended that clinicians should choose the method that best fits their personal preference, the patient population served and the practice setting (U.S. Preventive Services Task Force 2002). NICE CG23 (2007b) does not recommend a specific tool for use in practice.

There are a number of patient rating scales that can be used for the patient to complete by themselves or with assistance. They vary considerably in length and content. NICE CG23 (2007) considered only three when compiling their guideline: Beck Depression Inventory (BDI), Hamilton Rating Scale for Depression (HRSD) and the Montgomery Asberg Depression Rating Scale (MADRS). Examples of others are listed below:

- The Hospital Anxiety and Depression Scale, has 90 per cent sensitivity and 86 per cent specificity at picking up depression when used in primary care (Zigmond and Snaith 1983).
- The Patient Health Questionnaire (PHQ-9) has been well validated as a screening tool for depression and is being used more frequently in practice because of its brevity: it takes approximately 2–3 minutes to complete (Ani *et al.* 2008). It was found to have 80 per cent sensitivity and 92 per cent specificity (Kroenke *et al.* 2001).

Websites for tools

- Beck Inventory of Depression (BDI) (this product is copyright to Pearson Assessment): www.neurotransmitter.net/depressionscales.html.
- Hamilton Rating Scale for Depression (HRSD) (no known restrictions on use): www.neurotransmitter.net/depressionscales.html.
- Hospital Anxiety and Depression Scale (HAD Scale) (copyright to GL Assessment): www.gl-assessment.co.uk/health_and_psychology/resources/hospital_anxiety_scale/hospital_anxiety_scale.asp.
- Montgomery Asberg Depression Rating Scale (MADRS) (must have permission from Royal College of Psychiatrists): www.neurotransmitter.net/depressionscales.html.
- Patient Health Questionnaire (PHQ-9): www.patient.co.uk.
- *Guide to Mental and Neurological Health in Primary Care* (WHO 2004): www.mentalneurologicalprimarycare.org.

Memory and attention

Mini-mental state examination

Some of the references for this section are quite dated as they are seminal texts and have not been improved upon since. They are all quoted in the more up-to-date literature.

For the detection of mild or early dementia the 6CIT Kingshill Version 2000 is now considered to outperform the MMSE (Brooke and Bullock 1999) but the MMSE is the one that is still most commonly used in practice. The MMSE is a well-validated tool and has a large pool of probability data and can be used to monitor progress of the disease, but it is very lengthy for use outside the specialist area and discriminates in the visually impaired and poorly educated (Wind *et al.* 1997). It takes 10–15 minutes to complete.

The **6CIT Kingshill Version 2000** (Brooke and Bullock 1999) takes 3–4 minutes to complete; it has a high sensitivity without compromising specificity and is easy to translate linguistically and culturally. The disadvantage is its scoring method which can be confusing but since its introduction onto computer software this has been simplified making it easier to use. To date it is backed by large population studies and does have good probability statistics.

The test pre-dating the 6CIT was the **Abbreviated Mental Test Score (AMTS)**. This test took only 3–5 minutes to score and was used widely, but its validity data are limited and it is now outdated. Like the MMSE it is not thought to be valid for the detection of mild or early dementia.

The MMSE, 6CIT and AMTS can all be found on www.patient.co.uk/showdoc/40002381/.

Clock drawing test

The use of the clock drawing test is supported by some for assessing some aspects of frontal lobe function and it complements the MMSE as a cognitive screening tool, but there is not sufficient evidence at present to suggest that it should be used as a stand-alone screening tool for Alzheimer's disease (Rao 2002). It is not included in the NICE guidelines for the recognition and diagnosis of dementia (NICE CG42 2006).

There does not appear to be a consensus in the literature regarding the superiority of the different scoring methods. One of the simplest forms of the test can be found at http://alzheimers.about.com/od/diagnosisissues/a/clock_test.htm.

REFLECTION ON PRACTICE

STEPPING OUTSIDE THE BOUNDARY

Lucy was referred to the Nurse Practitioner (NP) by the General Practitioner (GP). She had recently moved to the area and had complex needs but did not want to discuss them with a man.

The GP suggested that she came for an assessment so that referral to the relevant agencies could be instigated. At the first meeting there was a frank discussion regarding the skills that the NP could offer. The consultation was difficult, as Lucy made little or no eye contact, the NP felt very nervous and defensive as she had never dealt with such an uncommunicative person before. The consultation was very factual and the NP informed Lucy that she would be referring her on to the relevant agencies once she had an understanding of the problems.

Lucy related her story briefly; she had been raped by a stranger when she was 5 days postnatal with her third child. She was going to the shop on the corner of her street pushing the pram when she was attacked.

Since then she has lost her children to the care of her ex-husband, been sectioned into a psychiatric hospital on two occasions and life was sometimes unbearable. This story was revealed over two consultations after which time the NP informed Lucy of the agencies that were available locally as she did not possess the skills that Lucy required.

Lucy pleaded with the NP to stick with her as she had been through all the specialist services and found no relief from her torment. She wanted to carry on seeing the NP as she felt that no one had ever listened before, they had all 'treated her'. The NP was completely out of her depth and was aware of this, which was a problem ethically for her as she did not feel that she could offer any form of therapy, advice or medication.

After much thought and discussion with colleagues, she sought supervision from a psychiatrically trained colleague, who encouraged her to continue with the case and offered supervision throughout. The NP discussed her inadequacies at length with Lucy telling her about the supervision and she was more than happy to continue seeing her.

Over the course of 3 months they worked together through her post-traumatic stress disorder under guidance and Lucy is now functioning at a more normal level. She now gets to see her children regularly and there is a chance that she could regain custody.

This story relates the importance of the therapeutic relationship we have with patients, even when we are not aware. Being aware of our competencies and limitations is critical. However, clinical practice is not always 'black and white' and we must endeavour to provide the best possible care to patients even in difficult circumstances. Lucy had a right to refuse the care that was recommended. It was decided in partnership with the NP that her 'best interests' were served by continuing care with the person whom she felt she could trust. This was carried out under close supervision after the community psychiatric nurse had checked that Lucy had full capacity to consent. Although the situation was not ideal, it was the only possible pathway that she was willing to accept. The therapeutic relationship that continued to develop between the patient and the practitioner was key to the improvement in health outcomes for Lucy.

CASE STUDY

A 36-year-old man presents requesting medication to 'make me feel better'. He was sent home from work as he was not concentrating on his work (drives fork lift truck) and he had an argument with a work mate.

He was reluctant to attend but his wife insisted. He had been feeling low for months and it was getting worse. He had been losing his temper a lot lately, he feels tired all the time, but also finds it hard to relax. His sleep is poor; he doesn't get off to sleep until 2–3 a.m. and then wakes early around 6 a.m. His social life has dwindled since having the children, as his wife works nights, mostly at the weekend. He doesn't enjoy his children and feels that he is shouting at them all the time (one aged

continued ➢

CASE STUDY *continued*

2 years and the other 6 years). He adds that he would never hurt them or harm himself, as he loves them too much. He admits that he has been very busy lately working on their new house and although it is hard work he is looking forward to when it is finished.

Past medical history: He has no physical symptoms and is otherwise in good health and there is no significant past medical history.

Test yourself

1 What are the salient points in his story?
2 What other examinations should be carried out?
3 What tools could be used to assist in his diagnosis?
4 What are the risks for this man?
5 What possible treatments could be offered?

Answers can be found at the back of the book (p. 127).

CASE STUDY ANSWERS

CHAPTER 1

1 • Nicotine staining (malignancy, chronic obstructive pulmonary disease [COPD])
  • Unilateral wasting of small muscles of hands (apical lung cancer)
  • Asterixis (hypercapnoea)
  • Pyrexia (infection, endocarditis)
  • Tachycardia (infection)
  • Dry, inflamed eyes (may be a sign of autoimmune disease involving the lungs)
  • Central cyanosis (hypoxia)
  • Lymphadenopathy (infection, malignancy)
2 It is not possible to tell from the history whether the increasing symptoms are due to respiratory or cardiac disease or both. Also consider mental health examination in view of possible depression due to his increasing symptoms and the recent death of his wife
3 Patient is taking atenolol. It does not appear to be achieving the appropriate reduction in blood pressure and may be causing the slow pulse rate, resulting in reduced cardiac output and fatigue. It may also be exacerbating COPD
4 May be one or several co-existing pathologies
  • Chronic uncontrolled hypertension causing onset of heart failure
  • Worsening COPD with heart failure
  • Ischaemic heart disease
  • Malignancy

CHAPTER 2

1 • Transient ischaemic attack (TIA): transient loss of power in limb
  • Space occupying lesion: transient loss of power, but unlikely as no other symptoms over the 3 days
  • Multiple sclerosis: transient loss of power in limb possible but in view of signs in preliminary examination the most likely cause is TIA
2 • Irregular tachycardia suggests atrial fibrillation, which could have precipitated emboli, causing TIA
  • Hypertension could precipitate haemorrhage, causing TIA
3 • Apical pulse and radial pulse to determine if atrial fibrillation or other arrhythmia
  • Full cardiac assessment to assess heart sounds, size and left ventricular dilatation or dysfunction
  • Bilateral pulses and blood pressure

- Assess for carotid bruits, but this should not be used in isolation for any diagnosis
- Electrocardiogram to assess heart rate, size and conduction ability
- Neurological examination to exclude neurological cause

4 • Admission to hospital for assessment (the risk of developing a stroke (cerebrovascular accident) after a hemispheric TIA can be as high as 20 per cent within the first month, with the greatest risk within the first 72 hours)
- Long-term management of atrial fibrillation (rate control, possible anticoagulation)
- Long-term management of blood pressure
- Further risk assessment: check blood glucose, lipids, blood disorders

CHAPTER 3

1 • Pulmonary embolus (must be excluded: patient has risk factors, including recent surgery, immobility)
- Unresolved infection/septicaemia
- Anxiety (recurrence with recent stress is possible)

2 Sweaty palms, tachycardia, tachypnoea, hypotension, pyrexia, low oxygen saturation, pleural rub, raised jugular venous pressure
Note the absence of any or all of these signs does not rule out a pulmonary embolus

3 • Cardiovascular examination to exclude cardiac cause
- Musculoskeletal examination, i.e. palpation of chest wall to assess for costochondritis (although tenderness to palpation cannot rule out an embolus)

CHAPTER 4

1 The patient is diabetic and it is essential to rule out a *Pseudomonas* infection. Although this is more common in an elderly, poorly controlled diabetic patient, it is important to consider as it may predispose to malignant otitis externa (usually caused by *Pseudomonas aeruginosa*)

2 An unsafe perforation

3 Cholesteatoma (requires urgent referral); primary otitis externa; otitis media with perforation and secondary otitis externa

4 Whispered voice test to determine reduced hearing in the affected ear

5 Diabetes, smoking, swimming. Long-term management of the patient should include smoking cessation and advice on ear protection for swimming

CHAPTER 5

1 • Acute or chronic viral hepatitis
- Tropical hepatotoxic viruses such as yellow fever
- Tropical hepatotoxic bacteria such as leptospirosis
- Protozoan infection such as malaria
- Helminths such as liver fluke
- Obstruction of the biliary system such as by a gallstone
- HIV/AIDS (human immunodeficiency virus/acquired immune deficiency syndrome)

- Primary or secondary carcinoma of the liver
- Liver cirrhosis
- Glandular fever
- Gastritis
- Drug- or alcohol-induced hepatic disease
- Underlying leukaemia
- Underlying or secondary anaemia

2 • Enlarged and possibly tender, hard or nodular liver
- Enlarged spleen
- Ascites
- Palpable lymph nodes
- Pyrexia
- Signs of anaemia such as pale mucous membranes, glossitis, angular cheilitis and koilonychia
- Spider naevi
- Palmar erythema
- Oedema
- Abdominal tenderness

3 Consider last monthly period and possible pregnancy as acute hepatic failure can develop rapidly following certain infections such as hepatitis E

CHAPTER 6

1 • Hydrocele
- Hernia
- Tumours
- Epididymo-orchitis
- Epididymal cyst
- Varicocele

2 **Hydrocele**: a fluid collection within the tunica vaginalis of the scrotum or along the spermatic cord; it is a non-tender cystic swelling. A hydrocele lies anterior to and below the testis and will transilluminate. The testicle should be easily defined unless the hydrocele is very large

Hernia: inguinal hernias may be associated with a hydrocele on the same side. When differentiating from an inguinoscrotal hernia, it is possible to get above a hydrocele on examination; bowel in the scrotum may transilluminate

Tumours of the testis or spermatic cord: testicular teratomas may present with a cystic mass that may transilluminate. Adults with testicular tumours may present with new-onset scrotal swelling which is attached to the testicle or cord; there is often a change in testicular size, shape or consistency. It is usually painless and non-tender on palpation

Epididymo-orchitis: there is usually scrotal erythema, pain and pyrexia. There is usually tenderness on palpation with a palpable swelling of the epididymis. A reactive hydrocele may occur in association with testicular infection

Epididymal cysts: these are well defined, fluid filled and will usually transilluminate. They lie posterior to and above the testis, within the epididymis, so the testicle is palpable separate from the cyst

Varicocele: this is an abnormal dilatation of the testicular veins in the pampiniform venous plexus caused by venous reflux. A varicocele typically feels like a 'bag of worms' and is more often left-sided (80–90 per cent, but 35–40 per cent are bilateral, rarely on the right side). The scrotum may be lower on the affected side. They increase with increase in abdominal pressure and are only palpable with the patient standing

3 Hydrocele

CHAPTER 7

1 Rotator cuff pathology – tendinopathy. Large tear is unlikely but small tear cannot be ruled out
2 Elevation against light resistance to demonstrate 'painful arc' may show pain in early abduction (between 60–120° if there is a rotator cuff lesion)
3 Advise simple analgesia, e.g. paracetamol (with codeine if necessary and tolerated). Physiotherapy may be equally helpful in the short term
4 Diabetes can be associated with adhesive capsulitis. When was this patient last monitored? Blood pressure needs urgent review. Needs dietary advice. Consider stopping ibuprofen as it may contribute to raised blood pressure. Smoking cessation should be encouraged
Discuss the patient's concerns regarding her employment and long-term prospects. Shoulder pain can become chronic and may affect her ability to work on the checkout

CHAPTER 8

1 Sciatica is likely in view of the symptoms, specifically the nature of the pain, radiation below the knee and associated paraesthesia. A thorough history is vital to rule out any 'red flags'
2 Root tension test, e.g. passive straight leg raising, may be positive. Crossover pain may also be elicited
3 Observation, palpation of the lumbar spine, assessment of the range of movement in the spine, evaluation of the neurological status of the lower limbs (there may be weakness or loss of tendon reflexes)
4 Likely non-pharmacological management: provision of written information and advice with the aim to promote a positive attitude. Advice to stay active and resume normal activity as soon as possible. Advice on appropriate lifting techniques and avoidance of heavy lifting. Assessment of patient's readiness to quit smoking and smoking cessation advice if appropriate. Prognosis: pain from acute sciatica usually settles within 6–12 weeks but in some people symptoms may persist for months and may recur

CHAPTER 9

1 • Plantar fasciitis
  • Morton's neuroma
  • Retrocalcaneal bursitis or Achilles tendonitis
  • Tarsal tunnel syndrome
  • Stress fracture of calcaneum
  • S1 radiculopathy
2 **Plantar fasciitis**: gradual onset, no history of injury, no inflammation, she is not systemically unwell and has no relevant past medical history. The pain of plantar fasciitis is often at its most severe during

the first few steps after prolonged inactivity, such as sleeping or sitting. Sitting with the foot elevated usually relieves the pain. For those who are on their feet all day, pain is worst at the end of the day

S1 radiculopathy or referred pain would usually have some pain in the leg also, very unusual to have pain in the foot alone

Morton's metatarsalgia: the pain usually starts in the ball of the foot and shoots into the affected toes. However, some people just have toe pain. There may also be burning and tingling of the toes. The symptoms are usually felt up the sides of the space between two toes. For example, if the nerve between the third and fourth metatarsal bones is affected, the symptoms will usually be felt up the right-hand side of the forth toe and up the left-hand side of the third toe. Some people describe the pain that they feel as like walking on a stone or a marble

Retrocalcaneal bursitis or **Achilles tendonitis** would have pain around the back of the heel rather than the sole

Tarsal tunnel syndrome has symptoms of tingling, burning or a sensation similar to an electrical shock, numbness and pain which is often shooting. This typically is felt on the inside of the ankle and/or on the bottom of the foot. In some people, a symptom may be isolated and occur in just one spot. In others, it may extend to the heel, arch, toes and even the calf

Stress fracture of calcaneum – the pain is felt in the heel rather than the sole of the foot

3 **Inspection**
- Abnormal arch height
- Absence of inflammation
- Absence of swelling
- Absence of bruising
- These exclude possibility of infection or gout or injury

Palpation
- Ankle joint tenderness: indicates or excludes stress fracture of the calcaneum or tarsal tunnel syndrome
- Achilles tendon: indicates or excludes retrocalcaneal bursitis or Achilles tendonitis
- Absence of joint tenderness, excludes joint involvement
- Application of pressure between the second and third, and third and fourth metatarsophalangeal joints – pain would indicate or exclude Morton's metatarsalgia
- Soft tissue tenderness alone is indicative of plantar fasciitis

Range of movement
- Abnormalities other than painful dorsiflexion, indicative of problems other than plantar fasciitis
- Straight leg raise abnormality indicates S1 radiculopathy; if negative it helps to exclude nerve compression
- Achilles reflex testing will help to exclude radiculopathy or neurological pathology if negative

CHAPTER 10

1 If there is a high risk of serious injury such as spinal fracture or cervical disc herniation. This would require immobilisation and immediate X-ray
2 Immobilisation and X-ray
3 Low risk

- Delayed onset of pain
- Low impact, low speed. The car did not roll over and the driver was not thrown from the vehicle
- Male under 65. Fit rugby player
- Ambulatory since accident
- Comfortable in a sitting position
- No neurological symptoms
- No other significant pathology
- No midline tenderness

4 Whiplash
5 Mental health. Possible anxiety, stress, low mood

CHAPTER 11

1 • The presenting complaint, family history and the fact that this patient is hypertensive, obese, black African, and an ex-smoker all point to a possible transient ischaemic attack
  • Other differential diagnoses include Bell's palsy secondary to otitis media, a space occupying lesion and multiple sclerosis
2 • Cranial nerve examination
  • Peripheral nervous system examination
  • Cardiovascular examination, including the peripheral pulses and auscultation of the carotid arteries
  • Examination of both ears
3 • Evidence of facial weakness (seventh cranial nerve). If the condition is transient there may be no residual weakness. In an upper motor neurone lesion such as a cerebrovascular accident or space occupying lesion, the weakness usually affects only the lower part of the face. In a lower motor neurone lesion such as Bell's palsy the weakness affects the whole of one side of the face
  • Evidence of a recent ear infection, which might precipitate Bell's palsy and vestibular dysfunction/loss of balance. Rinne and Webber tests to assess for conductive/sensorineural hearing impairment. Conductive deafness may be due to past surgery or a recent ear infection. It would be useful to compare with the results of old hearing tests if available. Evidence of sensorineural deafness might suggest a cranial nerve lesion
  • Evidence of other cranial nerve dysfunction. Cranial nerves 3, 5, 6, 7 and 8 in particular may be involved in multiple sclerosis
  • Problems with gait/balance point to an upper motor neurone lesion or a vestibular disorder
  • Increased tone, and reflexes on the right might point to an upper motor neurone lesion such as a cerebrovascular accident or space occupying lesion
  • Atrial fibrillation might precipitate a cerebrovascular accident
  • Carotid bruits and absence/reduction in peripheral pulses are indicative of arterial atheroma and possible subsequent cerebrovascular accident

CHAPTER 12

1 Corneal ulcer, abrasion, foreign body, keratitis, iritis and acute glaucoma
2 Red eye and whether unilateral or bilateral, ciliary flush, cloudy cornea, distinct corneal opacity, discharge and if so the type of discharge, irregular pupil, fixed semi-dilated pupil, hardness of the

globe, hypopyon, foreign body, epiphoria, rash

3 Stain with fluorescein and examine with a colbalt blue light/slit lamp

4 • Wearing of contact lenses is associated with infection. Pseudomonas in particular could predispose to keratitis

 • Diving, flying, and dry eyes precipitated by diannette, could compromise the integrity of the corneal surface

 • Sunlight could trigger herpes

 • A family history of autoimmune disease could predispose to iritis and therefore acute glaucoma

 • Myopia predisposes to glaucoma

 • Anaemia, travelling across time zones, and possible dehydration from heat and alcohol could lower resistance to infection

CHAPTER 13

1 • Low mood,

 • Lack of energy, feeling tired all the time

 • Inability to relax

 • Sleep pattern disturbed

 • Lack of concentration

 • These symptoms are included in the World Health Organization (WHO) symptoms list for diagnosis of depression

2 • A physical cause for his symptoms must be ruled out. A full preliminary examination should be carried out

 • Further examination will be guided according to findings of preliminary examination, e.g. cardiac if hypertensive or tachycardic, abdominal examination if drinking heavily, respiratory if smoking

 • Full blood screen, e.g. full blood count, thyroid function, liver function test, renal screen, blood glucose

3 There should be five symptoms present for the diagnosis to be confirmed (WHO checklist). The additional use of any of the tools listed will help to monitor the effects of treatment, e.g. HAD scale, PHQ-9, HRSD, BDI or MADRS

4 He is not in danger; he has already admitted that he would not consider harming himself or others, but if he continues with his current situation, his condition may deteriorate

5 Watch and wait: this is a mild/moderate depression, more than likely precipitated by his current busy lifestyle. Discussion around modification of current lifestyle is essential, allowing more time for his relationship with his wife and time for recreation, which is not currently happening. No need for medication at this present time and this should be explained to the patient, with a clear plan for review and monitoring

REFERENCES

Albers P, Albrecht W, Algaba F, Bokemeyer C, Cohn-Cedermark G, Fizazi A, Horwich A, Laguna M (2009) Guidelines on testicular cancer, European Association of Urology. www.uroweb.org/fileadmin/tx_eauguidelines/2009/Full/Testis_Cancer.pdf (Accessed 12/9/09).

Alshehri M, Ibrahim A, Abuaisha N, Malatani T, Abu-Eshy S, Khairulla S, Bahamdan K (1995) Value of rebound tenderness in acute appendicitis. *East Afr Med J* 72(8):504–6.

Anderson N, Mason D, Fink J, Bergin P, Charleston A, Gamble G (2005) Detection of focal cerebral hemisphere lesions using the neurological examination. *J Neurol Neurosurg Psychiatry* 76(4):545–9.

Andersson R, Hugander A, Ghazi S, Ravn H, Offenbartl S, Nyström P, Olaison G (2000) Why does the clinical diagnosis fail in suspected appendicitis? *Eur J Surg* 166(10):796–802.

Ang C, Dawson R, Hall C, Farmer M (2008) The diagnostic value of digital rectal examination in primary care for palpable rectal tumour. *Colorectal Dis* 10(8):789–92.

Ani C, Bazargan M, Hindman D, Bell D, Farooq M, Akhanjee L, Yemofio F, Baker R, Rodriguez M (2008) Depression symptomatology and diagnosis: discordance between patients and physicians in primary care settings. *BMC Fam Pract* 9:1.

Arroll B, Khin N, Kerse N (2003) Screening for depression in primary care with two verbally asked questions: cross sectional study. *BMJ* 327(7424):1144–6.

Austoker J (1994) Cancer prevention in primary care: screening for ovarian, prostatic and testicular cancers. *BMJ* 309(6950):315–20.

Babu A, Kymes S, Carpenter Fryer S (2003) Eponyms and the diagnosis of aortic regurgitation: what says the evidence? *Ann Intern Med* 138(9):736–42.

Bagai A, Thavendiranathan P, Detsky A (2006) Does this patient have a hearing impairment? *JAMA* 295(4):416–28.

Barkun A, Camus M, Meagher T, Green L, Coupal L, De Stempel J, Grover A (1989) Splenic enlargement and Traube's space: how useful is percussion? *Am J Med* 87(5):562–6.

Barkun A, Camus M, Meagher T, Green L, Coupal L, De Stempel J, Grover S (1991) The bedside assessment of splenic enlargement. *Am J Med* 91(5):512–8.

Bass S, Cooper J, Feldman J, Horn D (2007) Comparison of an automated confrontation testing device versus finger counting in the detection of field loss. *Optometry* 78(8):390–5.

Bogduk N, McGuirk B (2002) *Medical Management of Acute and Chronic Low Back Pain. An Evidence Based Approach.* Elsevier: Amsterdam.

British Hypertension Society (2008) Automatic digital blood pressure devices for clinical use and also suitable for home/self. www.bhsoc.org/bp_monitors/automatic.stm (Accessed 6/9/08).

British Thoracic Society (2001) Guidelines for the management of community acquired pneumonia in adults. *Thorax* 56(Suppl 4): iv 1–64. http://thorax.bmj.com/cgi/reprint/56/suppl_4/iv1 (Accessed 9/3/09).

Brooke P, Bullock R (1999) Validation of a 6 item cognitive impairment test with a view to primary care usage. *Int J Geriatr Psychiatry* 14(11):936–40.

Brown T, Herbert M (2003) Medical myth: bimanual pelvic examination is a reliable decision aid in the investigation of acute abdominal pain or vaginal bleeding. *CJEM* 5(2):120–2.

Calis M, Akgün K, Birtane M, Karacan I, Calis H, Tüzün F (2000) Diagnostic values of clinical diagnostic tests in subacromial impingement syndrome. *Ann Rheum Dis* 59(1): 44–7.

Centor R, Whitherspoon J, Dalton H, Brody C, Link K (1981) The diagnosis of strep throat in adults in the emergency room. *Med Decis Making* 1(3):239–46.

Chang Y, Jeong Y, Ko B (2008) A case of an asymptomatic intralenticular foreign body. *Korean J Ophthalmol* 22(4):272–5.

Chong C, Street P (2008) Pneumonia in the elderly: a review of the epidemiology, pathogenesis, microbiology, and clinical features. *South Med J* 101(11):1141–5 www.sma.org/pdfs/objecttypes/smj/B541CB67–1109-A387–609 C39042C7490C1/1141.pdf (Accessed 9/3/09).

Chongtham D, Singh M, Kalantri S, Pathak S (1997a) Accuracy of palpation and percussion manoeuvres in the diagnoses of splenomegaly. *Indian J Med Sci* 51(11):409–16.

Chongtham D, Singh M, Kalantri S, Pathak S (1997b) A simple bedside manoeuvre to detect ascites. *Natl Med J India* 10(1):13–4.

Chongtham D, Singh M, Kalantri S, Pathak S, Jain A (1998) Accuracy of clinical manoeuvres in detection of minimal ascites. Indian *J Med Sci* 52(11):514–20.

Choudhry N, Etchells E (1999) The rational clinical examination. Does this patient have aortic regurgitation? *JAMA* 281(23):2231–8.

Cibere J, Thorne A, Bellamy N, Greidanus N, Chalmers A, Mahomed N, Shojania K, Kopec J, Esdaile J (2008) Reliability of the hip examination in osteoarthritis: effect of standardization. *Arthritis Res* 59(3):373–381.

Close R, Sachs C, Dyne P (2001) Reliability of bimanual pelvic examinations performed in emergency departments. *West J Med* 175(4):240–244.

Costa L, Maraschin J, Xavier de Castro J, Gross J, Friedman, R (2006) A simplified protocol to screen for distal polyneuropathy in type 2 diabetic patients. *Diabetes Res Clin Pract* 73(3):292–7.

Cretikos M, Bellomo R, Hillman K, Chen J, Finfer S, Flabouris A (2008) Respiratory rate: the neglected vital sign. *Med J Australia* 188(11):657–9.

Croft P (2000) Is life becoming more of a pain. *Student BMJ* 8:217–258 http://archive.student.bmj.com/issues/ 00/07/editorials/220.php (Accessed 28/8/08).

Dalton J, Robinson J (2001) Palpable purpura on the extremities. *Arch Dermatol* 137(7):957–62.

D'Arcy C, McGee S (2000) The rational clinical examination. Does this patient have carpal tunnel syndrome? *JAMA* 283(23):3110–17.

Daniels I, Layer G (2003) Testicular tumours presenting as gynaecomastia. *Eur J Surg Oncol* 29(5):437–9.

Davis E (2002) Clinical examination of the knee following trauma: an evidence-based perspective. *Trauma* 4(3):135–45.

D'Costa H, George G, Parry M, Pullinger R, Skinner D, Thomas S, Todd B, Wilson M (2005) Pitfalls in the clinical diagnosis of vertebral fractures: a case series in which posterior midline tenderness was absent. *Emerg Med J* 22(5):330–2.

Del Mar C, Glasziou P, Spinks A (2004) Antibiotics for sore throat. *Cochrane Database Syst Rev.* 2:CD000023.

Department of Health (2001) Good practice in consent implementation guide: consent to examination or treatment. London: Crown copyright.

Devillé W, van der Windt D, Dzaferagić A, Bezemer P, Bouter L (2000) The test of Lasègue: systematic review of the accuracy in diagnosing herniated discs. *Spine* (Phila Pa 1976) 25(9):1140–7.

Dragisic K, Padilla L, Milad M (2003) The accuracy of the rectovaginal examination in detecting cul-de-sac disease in patients under general anaesthesia. *Hum Reprod* 18(8):1712–15.

Draper R (2008) Heart auscultation. www.patient.co.uk/showdoc/40000504/ (Accessed 7/4/09).

Drazner M, Rame J, Stevenson L, Dries D (2001) Prognostic importance of elevated jugular venous pressure and a third heart sound in patients with heart failure. *N Engl J Med* 345(8):574–81.

Duane T, Dechert T, Wolfe L, Aboutanos M, Malhotra M, Ivatury R (2007) Clinical examination and its reliability in identifying cervical spine fractures. *J Trauma* 62(6):1405–8.

Dubey S, Swaroop A, Jain R, Verma K, Garg P, Agarwal S (2000) Percussion of Traube's space: a useful index of splenic enlargement. *J Assoc Physicians India* 48(3):326–8.

EMIS Mentor Authoring Team (2007) Spinal disc problems (including red flag signs). www.patient.co.uk/showdoc/40025967 (Accessed 12/8/08).

Eskelinen M, Ikonen J, Lipponen P (1994) Contributions of history-taking, physical examination, and computer assistance to diagnosis of acute small-bowel obstruction. A prospective study of 1333 patients with acute abdominal pain. *Scand J Gastroenterol* 29(8):715–21.

European Association of Urology. *Guidelines on testicular cancer.* (2008) The Netherlands: EAU. www.guideline.gov/summary/summary.aspx?doc_id=12525 (Accessed 8/4/09).

Fernández A, Sorokin A, Thompson P (2007) Corneal arcus as coronary artery disease risk factor. *Atherosclerosis* 193(2):235–40.

Fink H, Lederle F, Roth C, Bowles C, Nelson D, Hass M (2000) The accuracy of physical examination to detect abdominal aortic aneurysm. *Arch Intern Med* 160(6):833–6.

Finlayson J, Kenmure A, Short D (1978) Cardiac signs for students: the wheat and the chaff. *BMJ* 1(6125):1471–3.

Frank C (2006) Evidence based checklists for objective structured clinical examinations. *BMJ* 333(7567):546–8.

Gade J, Kruse P, Anderson O, Pedersen S, Boesby S (1998) Physicians' abdominal auscultation. A multi-rater agreement study. *Scand J Gastroenterol* 33(7):773–7.

Gilbert V (1994) Detection of the liver below the costal margin: comparative value of palpation, light percussion, and auscultatory percussion. *South Med J* 87(2):182–6.

Gill G, Cole D, Lebowitz H, Diamond J (2004) Accuracy of screening for diabetic retinopathy by family physicians. *Ann Fam Med* 2(3):218–20.

Gokula R, Khasnis A (2003) Asterixis. *J Postgrad Med* 49(3):272–5.

Golledge J, Toms A, Franklin I, Scriven M, Galland R (1996) Assessment of peritonism in appendicitis. *Ann R Coll Surg Engl* 78(1):11–4.

Gonzalez R, Fried P, Bukhalo M, Holevar M, Falimirski M (1999) Role of clinical examination in screening for blunt cervical spine injury. *J Am Coll Surg* 189(2):152–7.

González del Pino J, Delgado-Martínez A, González González I, Lovic A (1997) Value of the carpal compression test in the diagnosis of carpal tunnel syndrome. *J Hand Surg Br* 22(1):38–41.

Goodacre S, Sutton A, Sampson F (2005) Meta-analysis: the value of clinical assessment in the diagnosis of deep venous thrombosis. *Ann Intern Med* 143(2):129–39.

Gordon-Bennett P, Ung T, Stephenson S, Hingorani M (2006) Misdiagnoses of angle closure glaucoma. *BMJ.* 333(7579):1157–8.

Gosselaar C, Roobol J, Roemeling S, Schröder F (2008) The role of digital rectal examination in subsequent visits in the European Randomized Study of Screening for Prostate Cancer (ERSPC), Rotterdam. *Eur Urol* 54(3):581–8.

gp-training.net (2006) *Examination of the Shoulder.* www/gp-training.net/rheum/exam/shoulder/shoulder.htm (Accessed 22/7/08).

gp-training.net (2009) The Back. www.gp-training.net/rheum/backpain/index.htm (Accessed 20/9/09).

Graff L, Russell J, Seashore J, Tate J, Elwell A, Prete M, Werdmann M, Maag R, Krivenko C, Radford M (2000) False-negative and false-positive errors in abdominal pain evaluation: failure to diagnose acute appendicitis and unnecessary surgery. *Acad Emerg Med* 7(11):1244–55.

Grover S, Barkun A, Sackett D (1993) The rational clinical examination. Does this patient have splenomegaly? *JAMA* 270(18):2218–21.

Gunson T, Oliver, G (2007) Osler's nodes and Janeway lesions. *Australas J Dermatol* 48(4):251–5.

Hansen M, Christensen P, Sindrup S, Olsen N, Kristensen O, Friis M (1994a) Inter-observer variation in the evaluation of neurologic signs: patient related factors. *J Neurol* 241(8):492–6.

Hansen M, Sindrup S, Christensen P, Olsen N, Kristensen O, Friis M (1994b) Interobserver variation in the evaluation of neurologic signs: observer dependent factors. *Acta Neurol Scand* 90(3):145–9.

Harkin H (2008) *The Primary Ear Care Centre: Guidance Document in Ear Care.* www.earcarecentre.com/protocols.htm (Accessed 24/8/08).

Heffernan D, Schermer C, Lu S (2005) What defines a distracting injury in cervical spine assessment? *J Trauma* 59(6):1396–9.

Hegedus E, Goode A, Campbell S, Morin A, Tamaddoni M, Moorman C 3rd, Cook C (2008) Physical examination tests of the shoulder: a systematic review with meta-analysis of individual tests. *Br J Sports Med* 42(2):80–92.

Hoberman A, Paradise J (2000) Acute otitis media: diagnosis and management in the year 2000. *Pediatr Ann* 29(10):609–20.

Hopstaken R, Butler C, Muris J, Knottnerus J, Kester A, Rinkens P, Dinant G (2006) Do clinical findings in lower respiratory tract infection help general practitioners prescribe antibiotics appropriately? An observational cohort study in general practice. *Fam Prac* 23(2):180–7.

Insall R, Davies R, Prout W (1989) Significance of Buerger's test in the assessment of lower limb ischaemia. *J R Soc Med* 82(12):729–31.

Issa M, Zasada W, Ward K, Hall J, Petros J, Ritenour C, Goodman M, Kleinbaum D, Mandel J, Marshall F (2006) The value of digital rectal examination as a predictor of prostate cancer diagnoses among United Stares veterans referred for prostate biopsy. Cancer *Detect Prev* 30(3):269–75.

Jackman A, Doty R (2005) Utility of a three-item smell identification test in detecting olfactory dysfunction. *Laryngoscope* 115(12):2209–12.

Jackson C, Glasson W (1998) Prevention of visual loss. Screening in general practice. *Aust Fam Physician* 27(3):150–3.

Jackson C, Hirst L, De Jong I, Smith N (2002) Can Australian general practitioners effectively screen for diabetic retinopathy? A pilot study. *BMC Fam Pract* 3:4.

Jackson J, O'Malley P, Kroenke K (2003) Evaluation of acute knee pain in primary care. *Ann Inter Med* 139(7):575–88.

Jepsen J, Laursen L, Hagert C, Kreiner S, Larsen A (2006a) Diagnostic accuracy of the neurological upper limb examination 1: inter-rater reproducibility of selected findings and patterns. *BMC Neurol* 6:8.

Jepsen J, Laursen L, Hagert C, Kreiner S, Larsen A (2006b) Diagnostic accuracy of the neurological upper limb examination II: relation to symptoms of patterns of findings. *BMC Neurol* 6:10.

Jepsen J, Laursen L, Larsen A, Hagert C (2004) Manual strength testing in 14 upper limb muscles: a study of inter-rater reliability. *Acta Orthop Scand* 75(4):442–8.

Johnson L, Baloh F (1991) The accuracy of confrontation visual field test in comparison with automated perimetry. *J Natl Med Assoc* 83(10):895–8.

Joshi R, Singh A, Jajoo N, Pai M, Kalantri S (2004) Accuracy and reliability of palpation and percussion for detecting hepatomegaly: a rural hospital-based study. *Indian J Gastroenterol* 23(5):171–4.

Joshua A, Celermajer D, Stockler M (2005) Beauty is in the eye of the examiner: reaching agreement about physical signs and their value. *Intern Med J* 35(3):178–87.

Kalantri S, Joshi R, Lokhande T, Singh A, Morgan M, Colford J, Pai M (2007) Accuracy and reliability of physical signs in the diagnosis of pleural effusion. *Respir Med* 101(3):431–8.

Karnath B (2003) Digital clubbing: a sign of underlying disease. *Hosp Physician* 39(8):25–27.

Khan N, Rahim S, Anand S, Simel D, Panju A (2006) Does the clinical examination predict lower extremity peripheral arterial disease? *JAMA* 295(5):536–46.

Kieling C, Rieder C, Silva A, Saute J, Cecchin C, Monte T, Jardim L (2008) A neurological examination score for the assessment of spinocerebellar ataxia 3 (SCA3). *Eur J Neurol* 15(4):371–6.

Kirby B, MacLeod K (2006) Clinical examination of the heart, clinical assessment. *Medicine* 34(4):123–8.

Kroenke K, Spitzer R, Williams J (2001) The PHQ-9: validity of a brief depression severity measure. *J Gen Intern Med* 16(9):606–13.

Lederle F, Simel D (1999) Does this patient have aortic aneurysm? *JAMA* 281(1):77–82.

Le Gal G, Testuz A, Righini M, Bounameaux H, Perrier A (2005) Reproduction of chest pain by palpation: diagnostic accuracy in suspected pulmonary embolism. *BMJ* 330(7489):452–3.

Leng G, Fowkes F (1992) The Edinburgh Claudication Questionnaire: an improved version of the WHO/Rose Questionnaire for use in epidemiological surveys. *J Clin Epidemiol* 45(10):1101–9.

Liddington M, Thomson W (1991) Rebound tenderness test. *Br J Surg* 78(7):795–6.

Linton S (2001) Occupational psychological factors increase the risk for back pain: a systematic review. *J. Occup Rehabilitation* 11(1):53–56.

Litaker D, Pioro M, El Bilbeisi H, Brems J (2000) Returning to the bedside: using the history and physical examination to identify rotator cuff tears. *J Am Geriatr Soc* 48(12):1633–7.

Littlewood C, May S (2007) Measurement of range of movement in the lumbar spine – what methods are valid? A systematic review. *Physiotherapy* 93(3):201–11.

Mangione S, (2001) Cardiac auscultatory skills of physicians-in-training: a comparison of three English-speaking countries. *Am J Med* 110(3):210–16.

Mangione S (2008) *Physical Diagnosis Secrets*, 2nd edn. Mosby: Philadelphia.

McAlister F, Straus S (2001) Measurement of blood pressure: an evidence based review. *BMJ* 322(7291):908–11.

McCullough G, Wertz R, Resenbek, J (2000) Inter and intra judge reliability of clinical examination of swallowing in adults. *Dysphagia* 15:58–67.

McGee S (1995) Percussion and physical diagnosis: separating myth from science. *Dis Mon* 41(10):641–92. www.ncbi.nlm.nih.gov/pubmed/7555568 (Accessed 25/8/08).

McGee S (2001) *Evidence-Based Physical Diagnosis*. Saunders: Philadelphia.

McGee S, Boyko, E (1998) Physical examination and chronic lower-extremity ischemia, a critical review. *Arch Intern Med* 158(12):1357–64.

McGraw P, Winn B, Whitaker D (1995) Reliability of the Snellen chart. *BMJ* 310(6993):1481–2.

McGuirk B, King W, Govind J, Lowry J, Bogduk N (2001) Safety, efficacy and cost effectiveness of evidence-based guidelines for the management of acute low back pain in primary care. *Spine (Phila Pa 1976)* 26(23):2615–22.

MeReC (2001) Specific issues in depression. National Prescribing Centre *MeReC Briefing* No. 17. www.npc.co.uk/ ebt/merec/cns/dementia/resources/merec_briefing_no17.pdf

MeReC (2006) Sore throat. MeReC Bulletin Vol 17 (3). www.npc.co.uk/MeReC_Bulletins/pdfs/Sore_throat_ Final.pdf (Accessed 20/8/08).

MeReC (2008) Routine use of antibiotics to prevent serious complications or URTIs is not justified. MeReC Extra No 31(January). www.npc.co.uk/MeReC_Extra/2008/no31_2007.html (Accessed 24/8/08).

Metlay J, Kapoor W, Fine M (1997) Does this patient have community-acquired pneumonia? Diagnosing pneumonia by history and physical examination. *JAMA* 278(17):1440–5.

Michel A, Kohlmann T, Raspe H (1997) The association between clinical findings on physical examination and self-reported back pain. Results of a population-based study. *Spine (Phila Pa 1976)* 22(3):296–303.

Mitchell C, Adebajo A, Hay E, Carr A (2005) Shoulder pain: diagnosis and management in primary care. *BMJ* 331(7525):1124–8.

Mol B, Hajenius P, Englesbel S, Ankum W, van der Veen F, Hemrika D, Bossuyt P (1999) Should patients who are suspected of having an ectopic pregnancy undergo physical examination? *Fertil Steril* 71(1):155–7.

Moses S (2008) Carpal tunnel syndrome aka: median neuropathy. *Family Practice Notebook* www.fpnotebook.com/ ortho/wrist/crpltnlsyndrm.htm (Accessed 9/8/08).

Mouth Cancer Foundation (2008) UK Statistics www.mouthcancerfoundation.org/ (Accessed 6/9/08).

Murphy R (2008) In defence of the stethoscope. *Respir Care* 53(3):355–69.

National Institute for Clinical Excellence (2006a) CG42 *Dementia: guidance*. www.nice.org.uk/guidance/index.jsp? action=download&o=30320 (Accessed 3/9/08).

National Institute for Clinical Excellence (2006b) CG34 *Hypertension. Management of adults in primary care.* (Pharmacological update of NICE Clinical Guideline 18). www.nice.org.uk/nicemedia/pdf/HypertensionGuide.pdf (Accessed 26/8/08).

National Institute for Clinical Excellence (2007a) CG22 *Anxiety: full guidance* (amended). www.nice.org.uk/ Guidance/CG22/Guidance/pdf/English. (Accessed 3/9/08).

National Institute for Clinical Excellence (2007b) CG23 *Depression: full guidance* (amended). www.nice.org.uk/ Guidance/CG23/Guidance/pdf/English (Accessed 3/9/08).

Naylor C (1994) The rational clinical examination. Physical examination of the liver. *JAMA.* 271(23):1859–65.

Nomden J, Slagers A, Bergman G, Winters J, Kropmans T, Dijkstra P (2009) Interobserver reliability of physical examination of shoulder girdle. *Man Ther* 14(2):152–9.

O'Donnell C, Elosua R (2008) Cardiovascular risk factors. Insights from Framingham Heart Study. *Rev Esp Cardiol* (English edition) 61(3):299–310.

Oluwole O, Odebode T, Komolafe M, Oluwole, O, Link H (2001) Effect of lower limb position on ankle jerk assessment. *J Neurol Neurosurg Psychiatry* 70(2):266–7.

Padilla L, Radosevich D, Milad M (2005) Limitations of the pelvic examination for evaluation of the female pelvic organs. *Int J Gynecol Obstet* 88(1):84–8.

Pandit J (1994) Testing acuity of vision in general practice: reaching recommended standard. *BMJ* 309(6966):1408.

Pandit R, Gales K, Griffiths P (2001) Effectiveness of testing visual fields by confrontation. *Lancet* 358(9290):1339–40.

Pedersen K, Carlsson P, Varenhorst E, Löfman O, Berglund K (1990). Screening for carcinoma of the prostate by digital rectal examination in a randomly selected population. *BMJ* 300(6731):1041–4.

Peeler J, Anderson J (2007) Reliability of the Thomas test for assessing range of motion about the hip. *Phys Ther Sport* 8(1):14–21.

Pines J, Uscher Pines L, Hall A, Hunter J, Srinivasan R, Ghaemmaghami C (2005) The interrater variation of ED abdominal examination findings in patients with acute abdominal pain. *Am J Emerg Med* 23(4):483–7.

Pirozzo S, Papinczak T, Glasziou P (2003) Whispered voice test for screening for hearing impairment in adults and children: systematic review. *BMJ* 327(7421):967.

Rao R (2002) Commentary on 2 clock test had high accuracy and naïve raters had acceptable accuracy for detecting dementia. *Evidence-Based Mental Health* 5:91 http://ebmh.bmj.com/cgi/content/full/5/3/91 (Accessed 3/9/08).

Rebain R, Baxter G, McDonough S (2002) A systematic review of the passive straight leg raising test as a diagnostic aid for low back pain (1989 to 2000). *Spine (Phila Pa 1976)* 27(17):E388–95.

Reichlin S, Dieterle T, Camli C, Leimenstoll B, Schoenenberger R, Martina B (2004) Initial clinical evaluation of cardiac systolic murmurs in the ED by noncardiologists. *Am J Emerg Med* 22(2):71–5.

Rice T, Rodriguez R, Light R (2006) The superior vena cava syndrome: clinical characteristics and evolving etiology. *Medicine* (Baltimore) 85(1):37–42.

Riddle D, Wells P (2004) Diagnosis of lower-extremity deep vein thrombosis in outpatients. *Phys Ther* 84(8):729–35.

Rovai D, Morales M, Di Bella G, De Nes M, Pingitore A, Lombardi M, Rossi G (2007) Clinical diagnosis of left ventricular dilatation and dysfunction in the age of technology. *Eur J Heart Fail* 9(6–7):723–9.

Saeed S, Body R (2007) Auscultating to diagnose pneumonia. *Emerg Med J.* 24(4):294–6.

Salerno D, Franzblau A, Werner R, Chung K, Schultz J, Becker M, Armstrong T (2000) Reliability of physical examination of the upper extremity among keyboard operators. *Am J Ind Med* 37(4):423–30.

Scottish Intercollegiate Guidelines Network (SIGN)(1998) *Management of testicular germ tumours.* No. 28. SIGN Secretariat, Royal College of Physicians: Edinburgh. www.sign.ac.uk/pdf/sign28.pdf (Accessed 12/9/09).

Scottish Intercollegiate Guidelines Network (SIGN) (2002) *Community management of lower respiratory tract infection in adults.* No. 59. SIGN Secretariat, Royal College of Physicians: Edinburgh. www.sign.ac.uk/pdf/sign59.pdf (Accessed 24/8/08).

Scottish Intercollegiate Guidelines Network (SIGN) (2003) *Diagnosis and management of childhood otitis media in primary care*. No. 66. SIGN Secretariat Royal College of Physicians: Edinburgh. www.sign.ac.uk/pdf/sign66.pdf (Accessed 20/8/08).

Scottish Intercollegiate Guidelines Network (SIGN) and British Thoracic Society (BTS) (2008) *British guideline on the management of asthma: a national clinical guideline*. No. 101. BTS: London; SIGN: Edinburgh. www.sign.ac.uk/pdf/sign101.pdf (Accessed 20/8/08).

Shahinfar S, Johnson L, Madsen R (1995) Confrontation visual field loss as a function of decibel sensitivity loss on automated static perimetry. Implications on the accuracy of confrontation visual field testing. *Ophthalmology* 102(6):872–7.

Sharma A, Machen K, Clarke B, Howard D (2006) Is undergraduate otorhinolaryngology teaching relevant to junior doctors working in accident and emergency departments? *J Laryngol Otol* 120(11):949–51.

Sheikh A, Hurwitz B (2005) Topical antibiotics for acute bacterial conjunctivitis: Cochrane systematic review and meta-analysis update. *Br J Gen Pract* 55(521):962–4.

Shelbourne K, Martini D, McCarroll J, VanMeter C (1995) Correlation of joint line tenderness and meniscal lesions in patients with acute anterior cruciate ligament tears. *Am J Sports Med* 23(2):166–9.

Sheth T, Choudhry N, Bowes M, Detsky A (1997) The relation of conjunctival pallor to the presence of anaemia. *J Gen Inten Med* 12(2):102–6.

Shub C (2003) Echocardiography or auscultation? How to evaluate systolic murmurs. *Can Fam Physician* 49(2):163–7.

Silva L, Andréu J, Muñoz P, Pastrana M, Millán I, Sanz J, Barbadillo C, Fernández-Castro M (2008) Accuracy of physical examination in subacromial impingement syndrome. *Rheumatology (Oxford)* 47(5):679–83.

Smith D, Catalona W (1995) Interexaminer variability of digital rectal examination in detecting prostate cancer. *Urology* 45(1):70–4.

Solomon D, Simel D, Bates D, Katz J, Schaffer J (2001) The rational clinical examination. Does this patient have a torn meniscus or ligament of the knee? Value of the physical examination. *JAMA* 286(13):1610–20.

Statham M, Sharma A, Pane A (2008) Misdiagnoses of acute eye diseases by primary care health providers: incidence and implications. *MJA* 189(7):402–4.

Stevenson J, Trojian T (2002) Evaluation of shoulder pain. *J Fam Practice* 51(7):605–11. www.jfponline.com (Accessed 20/07/08).

Stewart R, Thistlethwiate J (2006) Routine pelvic examination for asymptomatic women – exploring the evidence. *Aust Fam Physician*. 35(11):873–7.

Talley N, O'Connor S (2006) *Clinical Examination. A Systematic Guide to Physical Diagnosis*, 5th edn. Churchill Livingstone: Edinburgh.

Tamayo S, Rickman L, Mathews W, Fullerton S, Bartok A, Warner J, Feigal D, Arnstein D, Callandar N, Lyche K, *et al.* (1993) Examiner dependence on physical diagnostic tests for the detection of splenomegaly: a prospective study with multiple observers. *J Gen Intern Med* 8(2):69–75.

Tholl U, Forstner K, Anlauf M (2004) Measuring blood pressure: pitfalls and recommendations. *Nephrol Dial Transplant* 19(4):766–70.

Tidy, C (2008) (For EMIS) Patient UK. *Hearing Tests* (Document Version 20 March 2008) www.patient.co.uk/showdoc/40000920/ (Accessed 20/8/08).

Tierney L, Henderson M (2005) *The Patient History: Evidence-Based Approach* (Lange Medical Books). New York: McGraw-Hill: New York.

United States Preventive Services Task Force (2002) Screening for depression. recommendations and rationale *Ann Intern Med* 136(10):760–4.

United States Preventative Services Task Force (2003) Screening for Colorectal Cancer: recommendations and rationale. *Internet J Gastroenterol* 2(1).

United States Preventive Services Task Force (2005) Screening for peripheral arterial disease: a brief evidence update for the U.S. Preventive Services Task Force. *AHRQ.* Pub No. 05–0583-B-EF August.

Uppal S, Diggle C, Carr I, Fishwick C, Ahmed M, Ibrahim G, Helliwell P, Latos-Bieleńska A, Phillips S, Markham A, Bennett C, Bonthron D (2008) Mutations in 15-hydroxyprostaglandin dehydrogenase cause primary hypertrophic osteoarthropathy. *Nat Genet* 40:(6)789–93.

Urbano F (2001) Homans' sign in the diagnosis of deep venous thrombosis. Review of clinical skills. *Hosp Physician* 37(3):22–24.

Urbano F, Carroll M (2000) Murphy's sign in cholecystitis. *Hosp Physician* 70(11):51–2.

Varenhorst E, Carlsson P, Capik E, Löfman O, Pedersen K (1992). Repeated screening for carcinoma of the prostate by digital rectal examination in a randomly selected population. *ACTA Oncol* 31(8):815–21.

Verma L, Prakash G, Tewari H, Gupta S, Murthy G, Sharma N (2003) Screening for diabetic retinopathy by non-ophthalmologists: an effective public health tool. *Acta Ophthalmol Scand* 81(4):373–7.

Welsby P, Parry G, Smith D (2003) The stethoscope: some preliminary investigations. *Postgrad Med J* 79(938):695–8.

Whooley M, Avins A, Miranda J, Browner W (1997) Case-finding instruments for depression. Two questions are as good as many. *J Gen Intern Med* 12(7):439–45.

Wilkins R, Dexter J, Murphy R Jr, DelBono E (1990) Lung sound nomenclature survey. *Chest* 98(4):886–9.

Williams J, Noël P, Cordes J, Ramirez G, Pignone M (2002). Is this patient clinically depressed? *JAMA* 287(9):1160–70.

Williams J, Simel D (1992) Does this patient have ascites? How to divine fluid in the abdomen. *JAMA* 267(19):2645–8.

Wind A, Schellevis F, Van Staveren G, Scholten R, Jonker C, Van Eijk J (1997) Limitations of the Mini-Mental State Examination in diagnosing dementia in general practice. *Int J Geriatr Psychiatry* 12(1):101–108.

Winters J, Sobel J, Groenier K, Arendzen J, Meyboom-de Jong B (1999) The long-term course of shoulder complaints: a prospective study in general practice. *Rheumatology (Oxford)* 38(2):160–3.

Woodhead M, Blasi F, Ewig S, Huchon G, Leven M, Ortqvist A, Schaberg T, Torres A, van der Heijden G, Verheij T (2005) Guidelines for the management of adult lower respiratory tract infections. *Eur Respir J* 26(6):1138–80.

World Health Organization (WHO) (2004) *Guide to mental and neurological health in primary care.* www.mentalneurologicalprimary-care.org/downloads/primary_care/Depression.pdf (Accessed 3/9/08).

Zech L, Hoeg J (2008) Correlating corneal arcus with atherosclerosis in familial hypercholesterolemia. *Lipids Health Dis* 7:7. www.lipidworld.com/content/7/1/7 (Accessed 8/3/09).

Zigmond A, Snaith R (1983) The Hospital Anxiety and Depression Scale. *Acta Psychiatr Scand* 67(6):361–70.

Zuhrie S, Brennan P, Meade T, Vickers M (1999) Clinical examination for abdominal aortic aneurysm in general practice: report from the Medical Research Council's General Practice Research Framework. *Br J Gen Pract* 49(446):731–2.

INDEX

Note: the page number suffix '*dis*' refers to topics dispersed through consecutive pages.